Rock, Meet Window

A Father-Son Story

JASON GOOD

CHRONICLE BOOKS

SAN FRANCISCO

For Dad

Library of Congress Cataloging-in-Publication Data available.

ISBN 978-1-4521-2922-8

Manufactured in China

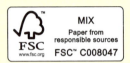

Designed by Jennifer Tolo Pierce

10 9 8 7 6 5 4 3 2

Chronicle Books LLC
680 Second Street
San Francisco, California 94107
www.chroniclebooks.com

Contents

Prologue

Thirty years ago, my father tried to force-feed me a beet.

We were sitting at the dining room table he purchased that morning in an auction at the Delaware County Library. After he struggled to get it through the front door, Mom had him place it just so and then spread an old blanket underneath. Armed with kitchen knives, Dad and I lay on our backs to scrape all the petrified Beech-Nut and Juicy Fruit off the bottom. We discovered that most of the gum was still soft in the middle, a little wet, even. "Maybe it's still good," Dad said, smiling.

We usually volunteered for disgusting jobs because they elicited accolades from Mom and accumulated the domestic capital needed to reject more menial household tasks. The risk of contracting typhus or the grippe from a gum-chewing schoolboy outweighed the mundanity of folding laundry or vacuuming the peanut shells we'd let collect under the sofa cushions.

But the library table wasn't the only source of excitement in the Good household. As a side dish to pork medallions, Dad made a new beet recipe, which he expected me to eat—a ridiculous presumption given that my diet was exclusive to shepherd's pie, various kinds of chips, and miniature microwavable sausage. No colorful fruits or vegetables touched my lips. Pomegranates looked like student art projects, pineapples were medieval weapons, and kiwis were nothing but limes that had been kicked around on a dirty barbershop floor.

These beets, bloodred and topped with a fresh mint leaf, belonged on a Christmas wreath, not inside my mouth. Dad polished off all three of his in less than a minute, and then, as he often did when tasting something unfathomably delicious, slapped his forehead.

"Jesus Christ, Jody, have you ever had a beet this good? Honestly, tell me. Have you ever tasted a beet *this good*?"

Under duress, Mom agreed, but added that they were "too rich to possibly eat more than one."

Unwilling to acknowledge that few things annoy a twelve-year-old boy more than the enthusiasm of his parents, Dad turned to me. "What about you, Jace?"

"They're disgusting," I said.

Dad said they weren't. I said they were. Mom left the room. And so it began.

He reached across the table with his fork, stabbed a beet from my plate, and held it in front of my face. "Just try it," he said.

"No way. It's gross."

"It's not *gross*. It's a beet."

"It looks like human flesh."

"Trust me, it's fantastic."

"No, it's not."

"You haven't even tasted it." He inched the fork closer to my lips. "Okay, just lick it."

"Lick it? Why are you so weird?" I swatted his hand away and tried to get up, but he stopped me and pressed the beet against my lips, causing it to slip off the fork and fall on the table. He picked it up with his fingers, mashed it against my mouth, and yelled, "EAT THE GOD-DAMN BEET, JASON!"

Dad could have opted for a gentler method like crushing the beets and sprinkling the dust over some Cool Ranch Doritos. But I know now that his frustration didn't have anything to do with food. After spending the afternoon figuring out how to tie an eight-foot-long, two-hundred-pound library table to the top of the family station wagon, and then taking heat from Mom for nicking the paint while trying to wedge it through the front door, he was tired and probably hadn't showered since the gum-scraping job. Add to that the enduring social and financial stresses of being an assistant professor of political science at a small liberal arts college (a middle-class Marxist in a *Hee Haw* town), and he was ready to blow.

And, yes, a rational adult would have acquiesced to Dad's demand, but children have no desire to avoid escalation, and the jaw is the strongest muscle in the human body. At battle's end, the color of Dad's hands matched my big red clown mouth. Together, we looked as if we'd been involved in a ritualistic animal sacrifice.

I recognized this as an opportunity to accrue some emotional capital and ran upstairs to collapse dramatically into my mother's arms. Within minutes, Dad joined us to apologize. His hands were still red, and they remained that way for days—as a branding of his offense. Not that he needed a reminder. A child's most valuable weapon, that which has kept all kids from being tried and convicted for crimes against humanity, has and will forever be the innate, near-effortless ability to elicit guilt and regret.

As a twelve-year-old boy, I assumed adult frustrations were mature, or at the very least directed at their source. I remember Dad calling the cable company because a football game had caused *60 Minutes* to start late for the third straight week. "Why the hell do they call it a two-minute warning when it lasts a fucking hour?" he yelled into the phone. Later that night, he became just as upset over the social injustices reported by Morley Safer. "I'll tell you what the problem is. These coal miners need a goddamn union!" Mom smiled, and I laughed at how ridiculously passionate he was.

Now I understand that Dad was merely venting his anger, the kind that all men carry around and release in their own dysfunctional ways. He was just a kid in grown-up clothes doing big-person stuff and trying not to punch himself in the face or intentionally drive off a cliff. I owe this enlightenment to becoming a grown-up kid myself: a state that's only been exacerbated by parenthood. I imagine Dad's days never quite went as planned. Mine seldom do. But it's impossible to address this frustration directly. Sometimes I scream into the innocent gray fabric of our sofa cushions when no one's looking. I haven't yet tried it, but I suppose yelling at a customer service representative from the cable company might do the trick, too.

With two young sons, Silas (five) and Arlo (three), my emotional life is ruled by the untenable condition of being hopelessly in love with tiny people who are too young to understand that they're slowly killing me. At no time has it been more important to be mature, and at no time in my adult life have I felt less capable. But I would never force-feed anything to a child. I'm a modern, enlightened father who deals with conflict in passive-aggressive ways that are likely far more damaging.

Silas will eat almost anything as long as it's exactly the right temperature. His acceptable threshold, however, is plus or minus five degrees Fahrenheit.

"*Too hot*," he'll say, pushing it away with an air of entitlement.

I dutifully blow on it and test the temperature with my tongue. "Okay, it should be better now."

"OW! It's really hot!"

"No, it's barely even warm."

"TOO HOT."

Feeling like a mere servant, a food cooler for his majesty, I blow on it *again*, only this time with a defeated gaze focused six inches above his head.

"Too hot," he responds, smirking.

And so it begins.

My visceral, human need in that moment is to take a forkful of the tepid rice and shove it in his mouth, but since that is no longer socially acceptable, I take the plate back and blow on it with the sarcasm of a teenage girl complimenting her father's dancing.

"Now it's cold," Silas argues.

"Then don't eat it!" I say and leave the room. When he starts crying, I realize I've taken it too far. Only one of us has a valid reason for acting like a five-year-old.

Though Dad and I responded differently, our behaviors came from the same well of parental frustration. We were frustrated that it took so much effort to control things; that fatherhood wasn't easier; that love, frustration, and fear can so easily blend together into a cocktail of angst. And yet, how is it possible that as stressful as family life is, we wouldn't change a thing about it?

Two years ago, himself many years removed from such parenting conflicts, Dad wanted to provide me with his own wisdom on fatherhood. He gave me a pocket-sized gift book called *Father to Son: Life Lessons on Raising a Boy*. Upon opening it, I was relieved to see that he'd annotated, crossed out, or corrected most of the "lessons." It was unlike him to promote pop wisdom. More than comedic ridicule (of which there was plenty), Dad's rewrites were his way of letting me know that he remembers, treasures, and has a sense of humor about our past.

> **Lesson:** "Be home for dinner."
> **Dad's revision:** "But don't ask him to eat beets!"

> **Lesson:** "Read to him nightly, he'll love it."
> **Dad's revision:** "He'll love it more if you make up stories where he's the main character."

> **Lesson:** "Give him responsibilities."
> **Dad's revision:** "Legitimate ones that he can handle and have some value to him."

But just as we entered the stage of our lives during which Dad and I could really understand each other—that period of confluence when he's not so old that he doesn't understand things, and I'm finally experienced enough to know who he is, who I am, and who we are—he started dying. The time we might have spent enjoying a mutual acknowledgment that we're grown-ass men with families, responsibilities, frustrations, anxieties, and flaws was shortened by a doctor's prognosis giving him nine months to live.

This is not a typical father-son tale. It is not about my dad and me scrambling to forge a relationship after decades of estrangement, or struggling to maintain one through a difficult time. As I see it now, this is the story of how a momentary alignment in perspective, coupled with a drastic change in the circumstances of our relationship, revealed that the epoxy in our bond is, for better or worse, professional-grade stuff.

I read recently that, as medicine improves, death is becoming more of a process than an event. We're often given ample warning that the end is near. "Pregrieving," or "anticipatory grieving," is common enough to have two names as well as various stages through which one can expect to pass. But like any kind of grief, be it anticipatory, chronic, delayed, prolonged, or distorted (apparently researchers' livelihoods depend on stratifying this emotion), no two people experience it the same way.

What we do with the weeks, months, or years depends on our relationship with that person and the circumstances of his or her illness. And so, the details and stories here are as idiosyncratic as anyone's in times like these. But sometimes it's within the specifics that we find common truths, and of course, sometimes we don't. Sometimes stories are just stories. I know in a few years I'll have a different perspective on all this. Then two years after that I'll have another, and two years after that I'll choke on a Twizzler and die inside a Walgreens. When you spend time with a person who has very little time left, it becomes clear that waiting to do anything only decreases the likelihood that you'll ever do it.

My memory of recent events is sharp and I'm in a fleeting state of lucidity, where connections between the past and present seem clear and simple. Most people couldn't write about this—their families wouldn't allow it. Fortunately, Dad loves being the center of attention, and he doesn't care why. If I'm quick, he might have a chance to read this. If he does, I hope he likes it.

Flight

Sitting on the kitchen floor, leaning against the dishwasher, my eyes drift in and out of focus as Arlo bangs on a drum set he's assembled out of pots and pans, while across the room his older brother, Silas, concocts a "potion" from face cream, baking soda, toothpaste, and I don't know what else. Maybe glue? Mouthwash? Mayonnaise? I've stopped paying attention. I love these guys.

A vibration in my back pocket startles me. It's a text message from Mom.

Mom
Call me—and get yourself alone—Dad's very sick. We need to talk to you.

I sit, motionless, staring at her words until they float on the screen. Heart attack? No, the tone is off. "Sick" means something else. Kidney problem? That's not "very sick."
Psychotic break? Maybe.
No, this has to be worse. Mom doesn't say "get yourself alone." But it is the dashes that really shake me. Why is it crucial for me to be alone?

I'm sure Dad gave her control over the wording of the text. He hates joint decision-making, opting instead to keep his desires private so he can complain about the end result.

I imagine Mom's index finger pecking at each letter as Dad checks the DVR for a new episode of the *Daily Show*. "Did you send it yet, Jody?" "Sent!" she responds, cheerfully so as to ease his anxiety.

A few days later I'll find a scrap of paper in her study with various drafts scribbled under the heading, "What to tell Jason." She chose the most alarming one.

I stand up, but my legs are weak and my head is tight. "Hey guys, just keep doing what you're doing. I have to run upstairs for a minute."

My wife, Lindsay, comes in. "What's wrong?"

"I'm not sure," I say. Without any real information, I'm stuck vibrating between fight or flight. Predictably, I choose both.

I jog upstairs into Silas's room and shut the door.

Mom answers on the first ring.

"Hi. Let me put you on speaker." She fumbles for a minute, accidentally mutes me, then puts me on hold. She fails even the smallest technological tests when Dad is watching. "Jesus, Jody. What did you do? Hang up on him?" Like me, he's loyal and caring, but fussy and impatient.

"Hello? You still there?" she asks.

"Yes, I'm here."

"Hey, Jace." Dad sounds calm, subdued: not himself.

"What's going on?" I ask.

Mom spits out the answer like it's burning a hole in her mouth.

"Dad has leukemia."

"Jesus. What?" I'd anticipated a stroke in his eighties, but leukemia? He's only sixty-eight.

There's a long silence. We've always been quietly intimate. As an only child, my parents and I developed an unspoken language long ago.

"This doesn't make any sense," I say.

"I know. That's how we feel, too," Mom replies.

"Obviously, I want to see you guys right away."

"Yes, come as soon as you can."

After another period of silence, we said good-bye. As I text with Mom for details, a piece of Silas's artwork catches my eye. *What is that? A giraffe? A dog with a really long neck? Wait, do I even know what a giraffe is? Or a dog? What does it MEAN that I can't tell animals apart?* This fear of going insane has driven me crazy for decades.

I walk to the top of the stairs. "Lindsay, can you come up here?"

"Right now?" she asks, sounding harried.

"Yes, please." I scurry into my office and sit. When she appears in the doorway, I tell her the news.

"Oh my God." She holds my head to her stomach, and I release the pent-up tears that men let fester because we're too weak to show weakness.

"Will he be okay?" she asks.

"No. His doctor says nine months."

"What? Nine months to live? Is he getting chemo or radiation or anything? I don't understand."

"My mom said something about chemo, but it won't cure him, and he might die while getting it."

"I'm so, so sorry." As she tries to process, the sounds of Arlo's frustration grow downstairs. Apparently, the seam on his sock has over-lapped his big toe. There's a special period in a young boy's life when, without much else to worry about, footwear ends up bearing the brunt of his angst.

"Shit. I'll be right back," she says.

When I can no longer hear the stairs creak, I put my head down on my desk. I'm blank, turned off, and though not the least bit hungry, I want to shove a cake in my face with my hands—a cheap white one with pink frosting like this woman I'd seen in a documentary about eating disorders.

I look back at my screen and see that the mail icon has turned blue.

From: Michael Good

Dear Jason,

I want you to know that I have no fear of death, none at all.
I have very little concern with what is in store for myself.
My first concern is with Jody, the absolute love of my life.
I deeply regret the burden this news will place on my family.

I'm not gone yet, but you need to know, that with this current
major exception, I would not change a thing about my last
68 years. Those years have been exciting, adventurous,
challenging and rewarding. They are so far beyond the dreams
I ever had for myself, that I consider myself beyond fortunate.

But most of all, you, Lindsay, Silas and Arlo make every other
adventure and reward trivial by comparison to the happiness
you bring me.

I love you all so much.

Dad

Sent from my iPad

So eloquent and concise, nothing unnecessary, nothing left out. When did he write this? I immediately consider drafting one myself for such an occasion, but decide it would be premature and in poor taste.

I yell down to Lindsay, "So, the first flight I can get is tomorrow morning at ten."

"Doesn't he want to see the boys?" she yells back.

"Good question. I'll ask him."

Jason
Should we all come?

Dad
Yes, that would be great, thanks. We know it's just so difficult for you guys to all fly out here.

Maybe Lindsay and I had complained too much about flying six hours from New Jersey to California with kids in tow. Of course we would all come. How bad do things have to get before Dad starts telling me what he wants?

I remember him and his siblings mocking their mother's passive-aggressive martyrdom. "Oh, don't worry about me. I'll just be over here dying," they'd joke. And now that he is doing the same thing, I wish I had brothers and sisters of my own. I imagine that in a few days we'd be sitting around a picnic table mimicking him: "I'm so sorry about this horrible thing I can't control that's making you all so completely miserable." We'd laugh, clink our bottles, and then stare off at people playing Frisbee nearby, squirming with guilt over having fun at his expense. I know that's trite, but as an only child I'm particularly vulnerable to advertising's mawkish portrayal of siblinghood.

This is my fault, though. I should have known Dad would want to see his grandsons. They're his Charlie Buckets, and he's their Grandpa Joe. "BooBoo," as Silas and Arlo call him, thinks kids should be allowed to do whatever the hell they want: "They've got a lifetime of stupid rules ahead of them." The boys eat pasta with their hands while sitting on his lap; play drums on his belly. He teaches them piano, and laughs when they sit on the keys. Not wanting to miss a single moment during visits, he tells them, "Now, when you wake up in the morning, the first thing you should do is come to our room and wake us up." I guess Dad trusts Lindsay and me to cover all the boring important stuff, like how to pet a cat *softly*.

On the flight to San Francisco, I'm still raw as hell. Is there a protocol for weeping on an airplane? Might this be an appropriate time to use my call button? Does the crew have a grieving curtain they can give me? There's an airsick bag for the physically ill. Shouldn't the emotionally ill have a similar option? A privacy mask? No. Crying with a mask on would terrify the other passengers.

My only option is the lavatory. Forced to choose between the mirror or the beige plastic wall, I go with the more self-indulgent option. *Oh, look how sad I am. This feels good. A damn ugly cry.* Between each wave, I fix my hair, wash my hands, brush flecks of dandruff from my shoulder. Finally, some *me* time. Other passengers are waiting, but my condition takes precedence over their pedestrian bowel needs.

In my seat, I'm distracted enough to hold it together for an hour at a time. The boys only know that BooBoo is "sick sick." I'm not sure what that means to them exactly, but they aren't crying, so I guess we did the right thing. Maybe death isn't an existential shit storm for kids. Silas watches TV and plows through multiple pouches of Delta Sky cookies and aside from complaining about the fit of his earphones every five minutes, he does quite well. Across the aisle, Arlo jumps up and down on his seat, squealing while the other passengers smile at him hesitantly, unsure if he's ridiculously happy or developmentally challenged. I try to distract him by playing "Walk up and down the aisles touching all the exit signs," but eventually he wants his mom. And his mom, like me, is busy faking a calm face and dreaming of parachutes. When we finally touch down, and the boys smell the stale air of Jetway freedom, excitement sets in for them.

Waiting for the Bay Area Rapid Transit (BART) at the airport, I'm holding it together.

I can do this. Maybe I can do this.

Silas and Arlo enjoy seeing how close they can stand to the edge of the platform.

"Stay behind the yellow line, guys," I say, calmly.

They ignore me. "Seriously, stand back. There's a train coming."

They don't listen.

"Silas! Arlo! STOP IT!" I'm yelling now.

They giggle and stand behind the yellow line, but test me by sneaking a foot over. Fear and frustration churn in my head. With a wry smile, Arlo looks at me and slowly scoots both of his feet over the line.

I raise my shoulder bag above my head and slam it on the platform.

"Stay the fuck away from the edge. Why won't you *listen to me*?!" I pick up the bag, planning to put it back on my shoulder, but instead I throw it down again.

"Goddammit! What the hell is wrong with you? Do you want to get hit by a train? Well, do you? *Do you?*"

"Do you want to get hit by *a fucking train?*"

My boys are afraid, and so are the Northern Californians in the station. This is an East Coast outburst. Lindsay takes the boys' hands as if guiding them away from a stranger who has asked if they want to see the inside of his van. "Daddy's having a tough time," she says. "We should leave him alone right now."

I stare straight ahead, defiant. My behavior was righteous and justified. When the train arrives, I get on, not caring if my family follows.

I sit alone, staring out the window. The fabric-covered seats on BART are all stained. In New York, subway car interiors are plastic and metal. Every night, they're cleaned with fire hoses. But San Francisco, apparently unwilling to acknowledge that people are disgusting, uses absorbent cloth for their seats. Thankfully, I resist the bizarre temptation to smell mine. I'd regained control of my actions. By the time we arrive at the San Leandro station, I'm crashing from the adrenaline rush and feeling calm.

From the top of the escalator, I can see them waiting for us outside the turnstile. Mom looks effortlessly glamorous, Audrey Hepburn-esque. Over the past few years she has started wearing her hair down instead of wrapping it up in a bun. Shoulder-length and almost completely white, it provides a nice frame for her Roman nose.

Dad looks the same, only vulnerable. He's slightly hunched, but that's nothing new; we come from a long line of tall people with weak backs. His hair is longer than normal: healthy, thick, and wavy. Still fifteen pounds overweight (all of it in his stomach), he looks like a potato that sprouted skinny arms and legs and a giant head. People mistake him for Bill Murray and Bill Clinton. Dad's thrilled with either. He's wearing his green suede jacket, black lace-up Vans, and the Levi's he gets in three-packs from Costco: the same thing he always wears when not teaching. It's strange, but perhaps I expected for a terminal illness to come with a new outfit.

Arlo and Silas run up to BooBoo and Mimi. Lindsay hugs Mom. Dad and I embrace last, and we make the most of it. Any traces of male hesitancy dissolve, replaced by uncomplicated, aggressive squeezing. "Careful, you'll crack my rib," he says. Twenty years ago, I snuck up from behind, wrapped my arms around him, and lifted him off the ground. He couldn't take a deep breath for three weeks. It wasn't my fault. I was young, and red wine had me feeling aggressively affectionate.

Dad insists on rolling one of our bags for the three-block walk back to the apartment. "Jesus Christ, I'm not dead yet. I can still roll a fucking suitcase." But a block in, I see he's fallen behind. "I just need to catch my breath," he says. I must look concerned because he seems conflicted. Not a tough guy, nor particularly proud, Dad likes that I'm empathetic, but he doesn't enjoy being on the receiving end of it.

"I'm winded because I'm anemic, Jason. Not that other thing." I suppose denial isn't bound to logic. Anemia is the prevailing symptom of his greater illness. His bone marrow creates bad blood cells that divide rapidly and never die. That goop deep inside Dad's bones that makes the blood which biologically connects me to him, him to his grandsons, and me to my sons, is spitting out a seedless fruit. That was the extent of what I knew about leukemia then. Hour upon hour of research later, I don't understand it much better. The Internet is a scary place: a Choose Your Own Adventure book that always ends in death.

Dad isn't interested in the specifics of his illness. I think he knows that, save a heart attack, stroke, bus accident, or environmental mishap, this disease will be his demise. He doesn't want to spend whatever time he has left hunched over a laptop reading medical papers and scanning the MarrowDisorders.org community forums. We won't go hang gliding, drive a convertible through Big Sur, or build a meth lab in the desert. Dad has no bucket list. His life, he once said, "has been one big bucket list." He's lived it exactly the way he wanted to.

The six of us cram into the elevator along with two suitcases and Silas's miniature rollie bag, which is probably filled with Pokémon cards, oven mitts, and one pair of shorts. The fluorescent lighting casts a slightly jaundiced light on the rest of us, but it's powerless against Dad's pallor. Normally a pinkish German-blooded hue, his face now almost matches his silver hair.

Arlo wants to push the elevator button. I can tell because he's jumping and screaming, "*Button!*" I pick him up, he lets out a theatrical grunt, and with a little undetected assistance from me, the button turns orange.

Mom grabs my free hand. "He looks pale, doesn't he?"

"I can hear you, Jody," Dad says. "We're in an elevator, for Christ's sake. Don't talk about me like I'm not here."

"You do look a little peaked," I say.

Silas looks up at me. "What's peaked?"

"It's another word for pale," Lindsay answers, putting an end to any further discussion of Dad's condition in front of the boys.

Mom and Dad's apartment is a long open penthouse with white walls and light blue carpeting, the kind of modest palace that makes baby boomers feel fancy and successful without appearing ostentatious. After a decade there, Mom is still tickled that the elevator button says "PH" instead of "5." The layout is perfect for young energetic kids. Our small Dutch Colonial in New Jersey doesn't provide much running room, but here the boys can gallop from end to end. It only takes a few minutes for them to find the Bozo the Clown Inflatable Bop Bag that Mom bought. It's a four-foot-tall punching bag, but people don't use the word "punch" around children these days. Bozo's big red nose squeaks when hit squarely, and he falls straight back only to pop right up again. Eventually, the boys wear themselves out, which is good, because Arlo napped on the train. Kids have a suspicious ability to stay awake during stressful events only to inconveniently crash when they're over.

Arlo has become nearly impossible to put to bed, routinely staying up until ten-thirty or eleven at night. At home, I sometimes take him to Whole Foods in his pajamas at eight-thirty to "run him." There's nothing cuter than a three-year-old sprinting through a grocery store in robot pajamas and shoes, and nothing quite as awkward as his six-foot-six father giving chase. Arlo is quick, reckless, and hard to catch, so I have to stay close. I don't want him knocking over a cheese display or falling headfirst into a giant barrel of quinoa.

Mom says I was the same way at that age. I never slowed down. To get me to eat she would place food around the house so I could snatch up fuel midstride. A piece of cheese on the corner of the coffee table, a cracker on the bannister, a slice of apple at the top of the stairs. The mice must have thought it was some kind of trick. "Jesus, these people aren't even *trying*."

In California, we have a time difference working in our favor, and after Bozo takes a standing eight count, and all the "Look how high I can jump" and "BooBoo, BooBoo, Mimi, Mimi, Mommy, Daddy . . . listen to me whistle!" activity is over, the boys wander off to yawn in private and pilfer from BooBoo's change bowl.

Silas's whistling ability *is* extraordinary, especially for his age. He reminds me of a snoozing Mickey Mouse from the 1930s: each exhale, the trill mating call of a sparrow. Dad is proud, too. The Goods come from fine whistling stock. "Yeah, don't encourage him unless you want tinnitus," I tell him.

He smiles. "Well, Jace, ya know what? One morning Silas will wake up and simply not whistle anymore. A few days will pass, and he'll forget he ever did. Believe me, you'll miss it."

He's right. Soon after an annoying habit disappears, we mourn it because change indicates the passage of time, and as much as we want our kids to be different in any given moment, we also want them to remain exactly the same.

The boys finally asleep, the four of us sit quietly for a while. Eventually Mom breaks the silence with a sledgehammer. "Oh, by the way, if one of us gets up and walks away, don't take it personally. We're just going somewhere to cry."

"We find it cathartic," Dad adds.

The moment is too morose for my family. We find the most abject sorrow to be innately comical. "Great, so we'll all be huddled in the bathrooms crying while Silas makes dinner," I say.

Mom laughs. "That's better than Arlo making it!"

"Yeah, I guess so . . . ," Dad mutters glumly, not playing along.

"Oh, shut up. We're going to have fun." I wasn't going to let him feel guilty about being sick.

Dad shakes it off. "You're right. Should we go to the city tomorrow? Or take the boys to the zoo?"

Mom looks nervous. "I think that's too much walking for you, Michael."

"We can rent you a Rascal, or a Jazzy, or whatever those things are called," I joke.

Dad hurls a pen at me and smiles. "Screw you."

"Who wants more wine? I know I do!" Mom seems relieved that we've moved on to levity.

Lindsay declines the offering. Dad feels that some rest might do him good, and I don't drink (though I used to and enjoyed it immensely).

"Okay, just me, then," Mom says, gliding off to the kitchen.

"I'll stay up with you," I tell her.

"Then it will be just us!" she says.

Trying to avoid talking about Dad, I get nostalgic. "Hey, do you still have my high school soccer jersey?"

"I think so. There's a box with a bunch of your stuff in the hallway closet."

"Remember how Dad would get kicked out of all my games for yelling at the refs?"

"Oh, it wasn't all of them."

"I can recall six without even trying."

"He didn't understand the rules."

"Yeah, and it was the referees' responsibility to teach him how offsides worked."

Mom laughed. "Of course it was!"

"I think that's why I started sucking on my jersey."

"You'd sucked all the blue dye out of the neckline."

"Sounds healthy."

"And if you weren't doing that, you were biting your fingernails."

"Dad always yelled at me from the stands."

"He did?"

"Yes, remember? 'Stop eating your hands!'"

"Oh God, I do remember that. You always yelled back, though."

Mom smiled and sipped her wine. "He liked it when you stood up for yourself."

"Yeah?"

"Uh-huh. It was something he never did to his dad."

"Yeah, well, he's a little less scary than Edwin."

The jersey is right where Mom said it would be, along with other pieces of memorabilia: a "book" I wrote in kindergarten, a wizard puppet Uncle Clement made me, some vintage puffy stickers, pictures from various graduations, and so on. There are also a few photographs of Dad and me from the early seventies. In one of them, he looks exhausted, slumped on a floral-patterned couch. His hair is long and greasy, clinging to the sides of his pockmarked face. There's a fat baby in light blue overalls and white pleather shoes sitting on his lap chewing a cork coaster.

"Jesus, look at this one. Dad looks like he was running guns for the IRA."

"I know! Menacing, right? He didn't always look like that."

"How old was he here? Twenty-eight or so?"

"Yes, you were eight months old, so he was twenty-eight, almost twenty-nine."

I see myself in the photograph, not as the baby, but as the father. We don't look particularly similar, Dad and I. I'm twelve years older now than he was then, have short hair, and the acne he passed down to me has lain dormant for years. What I recognize is a state of mental fuzziness that fathers have after fully understanding they can't turn back, and wouldn't even if they could.

It seems impossible that forty years could simply evaporate. He was so young then. But I realize that what happened in that time was me. Salt-and-pepper hair and reading glasses, *shit, I'm old now, too.*

"I want to show this stuff to Silas," I say.

"Okay, sounds good. I'm heading off to bed."

"Me, too. See you in the morning. I love you."

"I love you, too." She smiles. "We'll get through this."

"I know."

I've seen pictures of Dad as a kid, standing with the rest of his family, all of them gussied up in their good clothes and forced smiles. I like to imagine that after church, or whatever the occasion was, Dad and his brothers went out for lime phosphates, played baseball until it got dark, and read *Mad* magazine inside their fort. On the way home maybe they spotted a dead body down in the creek bed. I want to believe that part of Dad's childhood was idyllic because the inside of his house was crowded, hot, loud, and tense: four children, two parents, and an invalid grandmother crammed into a tiny three-bedroom ranch.

Dad's father, Edwin, worked at a factory in Dayton, Ohio, that made, as he put it, "tools people use to fix airplanes or some shit." He was a bitter patriarch who, according to legend, wasn't even ticklish. His calloused hands, ripped forearms, and greased-back hair were matched with a smoldering depression fueled by disappointment that his sons didn't share his interests in fishing and wildlife. Instead, Dad wanted acting and dancing lessons. Considering that Edwin wouldn't let his sons ride the bench on the carousel because it was "for fairies and cripples," I'm surprised Dad had the nerve to ask for tap shoes.

I went fishing with Edwin maybe a dozen times. Once, for reasons I can't remember, he had to drive us to the river in Mom and Dad's station wagon. Sitting in the passenger seat, with the car still in front of our house, I watched as he jammed "the shifter" down and pulled it back, calling it a "motherfucker" and a "goddamn piece of shit." The car lurched forward, backward, then coughed and stalled. He fiddled with the key, revved the engine, and tried again, but got the same result. "Piece of shit car," he said, too proud to admit he'd never learned to operate a manual transmission.

Eventually, we sputtered our way to the bait store, bought a foam cup full of night crawlers, then sputtered to the river. With Edwin still hot and embarrassed, we stood in silence, staring at two motionless bobbers for an hour. I was afraid to talk to him, and he didn't know how to talk to me. But we knew this about each other, and since neither of us made any awkward efforts to converse, we enjoyed our quiet time, just being. I think that's what he always wanted: quiet.

When it was time to leave, Edwin couldn't figure out how to put the station wagon in reverse. Fed up, he stepped on the gas and jammed the car into first gear. With the tires spinning, he made an angry, grass-ruining U-turn out of the parking lot. When we got back to the house, Edwin let Dad know that his "goddamn car was broken."

After a mostly brutish life, Edwin retired on the very day he was eligible and spent his remaining years lying on the sofa. If any of us inquired as to his plans, he'd snap, "*Nothing*. That's my plan! I'm doin' NOTHIN'." His mind quickly deteriorated into dementia. He'd spent the previous forty years watching in disbelief as his first son became a professor, his second an artist, and his third, a musician. A fourth son surely would have become a massage therapist. Perhaps the best way to guide a child toward something is to ridicule it.

I was in my early twenties when he died. After his funeral, the family congregated at my grandmother's house. I'd never spoken much to Walt (Edwin's youngest brother and doppelgänger) but as Walt was leaving, he found me, shook my hand, looked me straight in the eyes, and said,

"Let's go fishin'." I felt as if a ghost passed through me. I don't think Walt intended to take me fishing, then or ever, and I likely wouldn't have accepted a serious offer. He said this, I suspect, as a way to remind me how much Edwin enjoyed our outings. He knew Edwin would never have told me. If I was feeling sad about his passing, this glimpse into his emotional life might have provided solace. Or Walt was drunk and I'm inserting profundity where there was none.

Later, after the extended family had left, I happened upon Edwin's life insurance policy on the kitchen counter, tucked under a tin of peanut butter cookies. It paid out eight hundred dollars: a sullen amount, though I'm sure my frugal grandmother made no complaints. With the addition of Social Security payments and a monthly stipend from Dad, she'd do just fine.

Not wanting to repeat the mistakes of his father, Dad steered me toward classical music and acting at a young age. Private cello, and then clarinet, lessons evolved into some more-than-gentle nudges that I try out for school plays.

In fifth grade, my stunning—dare I say genre-redefining— portrayal of the caterpillar in *James and the Giant Peach* got the attention of Bo Rabby, the theater director at Ohio Wesleyan University. His daughter was in the play, too, and she made for a damn fine ladybug. Later, Bo told Dad that I'd be perfect for the role of Howard in an upcoming university production of *Inherit the Wind*, a play about the first legal case defending the constitutionality of teaching evolution in public schools. Without first asking me if I was interested, Dad told Bo I'd be thrilled to do it. When I agreed, he celebrated like a mother whose son had been drafted in the first round by the Lakers. This wasn't only an unrealized childhood dream of his but also a political topic in which he had a fiery passion. Dad came to every rehearsal, befriended the whole cast, knew all my lines, and then when opening night finally came, he spent it in the bathroom of the Chapelier Theater vomiting his nerves into a toilet bowl.

Dad was hesitant to push too hard. Perhaps he knew that would only send me in the opposite direction. When I turned down the role of George in a local production of *Our Town* because I wanted to attend soccer camp, he smiled, nodded, and then probably sequestered himself in the basement to scream into a stack of oily rags or squeeze his head in a vise. Despite being disappointed, he wanted my world to be open. Forcing me into music or acting would have been the other side—an opposite, equal, and arguably better side—of his father not letting him ride the bench on a carousel.

Dad's desire for his progeny to grow up free-range has only increased since becoming a grandfather. The advice book he gave me says a lot about education. Dad crossed out all of it and wrote, DON'T SEND THEM TO SCHOOL!

Clearly, Dad would prefer that Lindsay and I homeschool Silas and Arlo. "Don't dump these precious minds into a broken system," he said. "Unless, of course, you want them to think in rote ways that contribute to the dominant paradigm." But since we aren't part of a traveling circus, and I don't know the difference between a porpoise and a dolphin (much less a buffalo and a bison), and Lindsay can only name four U.S. presidents, we figured traditional school teamed with frequent visits to the alternative learning house of BooBoo might be a safer bet.

Perhaps it was my failures in school that turned him against formal education. I was always a horrible student: distracted, antsy, disruptive. After trying everything else, Mom and Dad bought a collection of VHS tapes called "Where There's a Will, There's an A." I rolled my eyes, and watched the first tape to appease them. Then I announced, "I know exactly how to get an A. It's the will that's the problem." This caught Dad off guard and he smiled. I think he took a little pride in my recalcitrance, but at that time, believed a good education was the only ticket to being a successfully recalcitrant adult.

Without any desire of my own to excel in school, Mom and Dad decided to force the issue by instituting a three-hour solitary study period in my room every day after school. Aware of how absurd this was, I followed only 50 percent of the rule. I hated missing out on all the after-school fun, like watching Barry Cast bite his arm until it bled, or avoiding Tim Fisher's Trans Am as it sped down "bus alley," but I was generally a good kid and tried to do as my parents asked. So I would come home, sit in my room for three hours, and stare at the wall. I found that more interesting than congruent triangles. It wasn't long before I started getting a little too brave.

I was in my room playing Atari with the sound off when Dad walked in. I knew I was in trouble, and I fumbled pathetically to hide the evidence, resulting in something out of a hackneyed Disney sitcom where I was reading a book upside down with a joystick in my hand.

"What the hell do you think you're doing in here?" he asked.

"Nothin'."

"Were you playing video games?"

"No."

"No? What's the joystick for?"

"Nothin'."

"Just one word answers, eh?"

"No."

This went on for long enough that he started preaching about how lucky I was to be allowed to go to school at all and other nonsense parents say despite promising themselves they never will.

I looked right through him.

"Are you even listening to me?" he asked.

"Nope."

He paused. Then in a soft, confused, and earnest voice, asked, "Why?"

"Because it's bullshit."

My answer hovered there for what felt like a full minute but was probably no more than a couple of seconds. I was waiting for some kind of punishment and assumed he was taking his time to weigh his disciplinary options. But to my surprise (and his), he laughed. He laughed hard—hard enough that I feared it was more of a maniacal laugh driven by insanity rather than amusement.

Years later, Dad said his reaction came from a realization that I was right: he was full of shit. The study-time rule was ridiculous, as was his defense of it, and I'd called him on it. I was now a man in his eyes, and though I would continue to be an idiot for another couple of decades, he spoke to me as an adult from that point forward.

Slightly Less Bad

The next morning, while the boys "help" Lindsay and Mom make pancakes, I see Dad in the bedroom, not yet dressed. He waves for me to come in.

"I want to give you something," he says.

"Oh jeez. Are we doing this already?"

He laughs, opens the top drawer of his dresser, and pulls out a pen case.

This makes three Montblanc pens he has given me over the past twenty years, each to commemorate the end of one chapter and the beginning of a new one. The first two he gave me when I was donning a cap and gown. I lost both. This one he gave me when we were both in our underwear, and I'll keep it forever. Or at least until Silas graduates from high school and has proven to me that he's mature enough to carry on the family tradition of losing it.

I'll give it to Silas, and he'll wonder, as I did at eighteen years old, why the hell his father is giving him a pen. He'll put it in his beat-up back-pack, slide into the passenger seat of his best friend's car, and they'll head off to a Grateful Dead concert, or whatever the equivalent of that might be in 2026. A few years later, I'll ask him, "Hey, whatever happened to that pen I gave you," and he'll lie, telling me that it's "somewhere in the apart-ment," and I'll pretend to believe him and try not to care that it's gone.

After Dad puts on his Levi's, Vans, and a navy blue T-shirt, we take pictures of him with his grandsons. They pose as requested, but neither of the boys has a good photo smile. Silas underdoes it and Arlo overdoes it, creating a digital memory of a sick man flanked on one side by ecstasy and on the other by melancholy. At home, Lindsay and I struggle to get candid shots of the boys. Somehow, the moment one of us pulls out an iPhone, they stop being sweet to each other, and we're left with a camera full of blurry action shots of Arlo in the midst of climbing on top of his brother. We often hide around corners and tiptoe from room to room. Our floors are creaky, so we slide in our stocking feet to avoid detection, but they almost always hear us coming.

The carpeting in my parents' apartment allows for easy stalking, and, eventually, we click off a couple of winners. Children miss things like fatigue and pallor, and we need to take advantage of that before Dad morphs into a gaunt bald man: an appearance even animals can't help but acknowledge.

We decide to take BART into downtown San Francisco to have lunch at the gourmet food court inside the Westfield shopping center. Dad likes the Korean barbecue counter, and we figure the kids might have some fun pounding on electronics at the various cell-phone kiosks. Dad feels strong after his small meal, so we head out onto busy Market Street. Across the way, at the base of Powell Street, is a Rice-a-Roni cable car, but the line of tourists in windbreakers makes it too daunting to consider. Silas points to it. "What's that train over there?" Dad jumps in. "It's a train no one's allowed to ride on."

"There's some shopping just up the hill," Mom offers. "I think there's an Urban Outfitters. Yay!"

"Oh, I wonder if they have the bed shorts I like. I need to replace mine," Lindsay says, as the rest of us wonder how one might wear out bed shorts.

I glance over at Dad for approval. "Yes, I can walk up the damn hill," he says. "Would you all stop worrying about me? Jesus Christ."

Lindsay shoots me her "I don't like it when your Dad talks like that" look.

After decades of practice, Mom and I have learned to endure Dad's acerbic quips by remaining calm and staring off into the middle distance, like dental patients during a cleaning. Tolerance pays off; these episodes are usually followed by spells of guilt, during which he offers to make coffee cake or change our water filters.

As we trudge past the white-shoed cable car hopefuls, the sun makes a rare appearance, providing just enough heat to release the aroma of San Francisco street piss. Arlo is already too tired to walk, so I scoop him onto my shoulders. Dad is struggling, too. Pale and winded, he leans against the side of a building, and then steadies himself by grabbing onto my elbow. We all hurry inside Urban Outfitters, where Dad sits on the wooden steps leading down to the men's department, head hanging between his legs like an NBA player catching his breath on the bench. Arlo, now suspiciously revitalized, takes off to join his brother, who is already fiddling with various products in the "Ironic Stuff from the Eighties" section.

I sit down next to Dad, but he's either too tired or too busy troubleshooting to acknowledge me. I want to tell him how tragically out of place he looks sitting next to a stack of "Naked Co-ed Rocket Party" T-shirts, but I know he's not in the mood. I have to get him the hell out of here.

After a few minutes, Mom and Lindsay appear with the bed shorts she wanted. The shrieking from across the store indicates that the boys have started fighting over what turns out to be an ABBA eight-track tape.

It's time to head home. Dad has no trouble walking downhill, but he falls asleep within minutes of boarding the train back to San Leandro.

When we return to the apartment, Dad's phone rings.

"Hello? Oh, hello, Dr. Levine," he says.

Mom, Lindsay, and I huddle around him. He waves us off, but we are undeterred.

After a torturous number of "Okays," "Uh-huhs," and "Thank-yous," Dad puts the phone down.

"Good news," he says. "Well, not good, but slightly less bad, I guess. I don't have to go in for chemo right away. My doctor looked at my blood and thinks my case is borderline. He'd rather treat me for this other condition called myelodysplasia." Dad pauses to catch his breath. "Honestly, I think he didn't believe I'd survive the other kind of chemo, so he's just going to give this a shot and keep his fingers crossed."

"Wait, so when do you start chemo, then?" Mom asks.

"He said in a few weeks. He also said that the prognosis isn't really any better for this condition than the other one."

"So still nine months?" I ask. "I don't understand that. What's the point?"

"But this new chemo won't kill you?" Mom seems hopeful.

"He says it won't." Dad pauses again, and I know what's coming next.

"Jesus, I'm really sorry I made you guys come out here like this. We really thought I might be dead in a week."

A few hours later, as I scrounge the makings of a sandwich, I hear Mom and Dad talking softly in their bedroom. Neither of them understands how loud their quiet voices are, and I've never told them. I've always been desperate to hear their secrets. I close the fridge gently and hear Dad say, "Well, this *is* my fault."

Mom appears in the kitchen and hands me a check for our plane tickets. "We're not accepting no for an answer." I slide it into my wallet and tell her that I'm coming back when Dad starts chemotherapy. She smiles. "Yes, that would be nice."

After three more days of playing, napping, laughing, and filling out online retirement documents, we have a plane to catch. Silas has to get back to school, Arlo misses his favorite cheese crackers, Lindsay needs the quasi-sanity of her routine, and I need some space, too. Knowing that I'll return by myself in the next couple of weeks makes the good-byes more tolerable. Dad doesn't like seeing his grandsons go, but thankfully we know he will be able to do it again.

Melanchoholic

At home. I feel off—disconnected from the world and everyone in it, including Dad. Waking up the first morning back, I'm uncomfortably aware of my own body. When I think of the blood in my veins, about my heart, brain, lungs, and bone marrow, I'm not struck by what a magical machine the human body is, but rather how it's designed to malfunction.

This is not a healthy path for me to wander. While in graduate school, I was convinced I was dying. Freckles were all melanomas. A sore neck was Lyme disease. Routine tinnitus? A common symptom of inoperable brain cancer. At the worst of it, a tingling sensation in my shins caused me to seek counsel from a neurologist, who was nice enough to send me home with the name of a psychiatrist. Now I fear that a fresh bout with hypochondria might become one of the emotional manifestations of my stress over Dad's illness. I'm anxious enough that my anxiety could trigger more anxiety, leading to a condition that is itself caused by anxiety. More than worrying about being sick, I'm worried about worrying about being sick. One might call this *tertiary anxiety*, or, more accurately, the pinnacle of narcissism.

I assume this all stems from my guilt over leaving California. Lindsay and the boys need me (I think), and Dad has Mom to care for him. Over the past few days, we've been texting and video chatting, but it's not the same. I can't sit next to him on the sofa and rest my head on his shoulder until it gets weird. I would ask them to move closer to us, but after a decade on the West Coast, they are convinced the New Jersey winters would kill them. They're delicate, tropical lizards: Mom the species that can only eat lettuce, Dad the kind that survives exclusively on unusual meats.

After finally settling into my old routine and accepting that my autonomic nervous system will likely continue to function for at least a few more years, I receive an email from Mom. She and Dad couldn't go to a movie the previous evening because the elevator in their building is broken, and Dad feared he wouldn't be able to climb the stairs back up to the apartment. I imagine them housebound: Mom reading, Dad catching up on episodes of his favorite crime drama while eating salami and intentionally breaking his laptop so he'd have to fix it. Had I been there, I would have encouraged him to try the stairs and helped him if needed. Mom can't do that. She's as old as he is. Though in good shape for her age, the idea of her providing any physical assistance is absurd, and Dad would refuse to put her in a dangerous situation, anyway. For years, it's been a running joke that they're afraid one of them might break a hip: "Don't fall off that step stool. You'll break a hip!" So sweet, sad, and accurate. A sixty-eight-year-old woman helping a sixty-eight-year-old man climb concrete stairs can only end in two ways: success or paramedics.

Feeling powerless and needy, I reach out to Jeremy, Todd, and Patrick: my best friends in high school. I wanted to connect with people who knew Dad *then*. Over the past thirty years, these three have seen Dad napping on the couch in his underwear enough to think of him as a second father. They would want to know what's going on.

I call Jeremy first, and somewhat disappointingly, he reacts as expected. He has always been emotionally inscrutable, especially with men. He was the only member of our youth group who opted out of the co-ed "cuddle puddles" during our biannual retreats to Camp Agape. Mom and Dad were reluctant to let me join this cult, but after seeing it was "ecumenical" (and would therefore technically embrace atheism), they gave their "blessing"—my pragmatism would be preserved. On the phone, Jeremy offers the proper condolences and support, but it's clear that he does so for my sake, as my friend. Dad's life doesn't have much significance to him apart from me, but that's not his fault. I appreciate his sympathy, but it isn't quite what I'm looking for.

Todd takes the news hard. I'm glad to see someone is finally living up to my ridiculous expectations. Todd spent his junior year of college with us in Florence, Italy: one of Dad's finer years. After soaking in the news, he says, "The old man will figure out a way to beat this. I'd like to talk to him, but only if he wants to. Have him call me if he does." I tell Dad later; he's touched but offers little indication that he'll call.

In first grade, Patrick and I appeared in a newspaper article together when our class made a ten-foot-tall papier-mâché T. rex. Over the next twelve years he was the guitar to my drums. Two inseparable boys in a band. As adults, we haven't kept in touch as well as we should have, and I don't want this to be the reason I talk to him for the first time in five years. So I text:

Jason
Hey man, I thought you'd want to know that my dad is very sick
with a kind of leukemia and has about nine months to live.

He responded quickly:

Patrick
That kind of took the wind out of me.

Jason
Sorry. I probably should have said hello first.

Patrick
Maybe. Shit. I know your dad as your dad, not as Professor Good.

Jason
Yeah, I like that. It's why you're one of the few people I've told.

Patrick
Damn man. Let me know if there's anything I can do.

Jason
Thanks. I will.

We have an idea of the age we might be when our fathers die, and it isn't forty-one. My grandparents died when Mom and Dad were sixty-some-things. I figured I would have at least twenty more years before facing this. Now I've forced my best friends to consider it for themselves.

Patrick tells his mother, who still lives in our old hometown of Delaware, Ohio. From there, the news metastasizes. I receive numerous Facebook messages from friends offering condolences and "prayers." Sickness is the new death in the age of social media. I thought this might frustrate Dad, but he has too much on his mind to care. "It's going to get out one way or another," he says. I imagine the hardest part of dying is everyone finding out.

When our neighbors in New Jersey ask about our sudden visit to California, I am met with some sad faces, but nothing feels real. Our block feels like a quaint, backlit movie set, and I am the only nonactor. I enjoy all the attention, but the gooey warmth of empathy isn't sticking.

Cori Lynn, who lives a few doors down, asks Lindsay how I'm doing. Lindsay tells her that I've been crying a lot, and this elicits another sad face, but I'm fairly certain women enjoy it when men cry. It helps them believe we're human.

In our small social circle, we are open about our mental health conditions and medications (we all know what each other is "on"). Cori Lynn suggests to Lindsay that I increase my Prozac dosage. I take her advice and am, predictably, stricken with diarrhea. It's uncomfortable enough to take my mind off Dad, though I don't think that's the effect she had in mind.

Cori Lynn's husband, Erik, recently lost his father to cancer. He's the consummate nice guy, always concerned with the emotional well-being of others, and I accept his offer to have a drink at the local pub. An enormous, six-foot-seven Norwegian with chiseled cheekbones and sunken, empathetic eyes, he picks me up in his Toyota Sienna, and I feel good, nurtured, like a babysitter getting a ride home.

At the pub, he orders a Guinness. I get an O'Doul's and wrap my hand around the label so no one can see it. There's a certain shame in being dry and Irish.

"Oh, I forgot you don't drink," Erik says.

"Now would be a great time to start again," I joke.

He stares. I'm often facetious with people who don't know me well enough to understand that I'm almost always facetious.

"That doesn't mean I'm going to."

"Oh, well, that's good, then. So how are you doing with all this?"

"Way worse than I would have thought."

Erik beams another dose of concern. His cavernous eye sockets cast small shadows across his cheekbones. Like most husbands and fathers our age, he's accustomed to consoling women and children, most of whom prefer understanding and listening over troubleshooting. His therapeutic gaze opens me up, and I tell him the story: the original diagnosis, the new diagnosis, Dad's current condition, and a few of the morbid, though humorous, anecdotes of our trip. Still, I feel ridiculous. Erik's father actually died, and mine has merely been penciled into the schedule.

"So, what kind of cancer did your dad have?" I ask, abruptly.

Erik soaks in my question and strokes his Disney-hero chin. His father's story is tragic: multiple remissions, an organ transplant, perilous fainting spells. All tallied, it was an eight-year process.

He orders another Guinness. My O'Doul's is still half full. There's no hurry with nonalcoholic brews.

Erik shifts the conversation back to me. "So, your dad had no symptoms?"

"None. They found it during a routine blood test for a kidney-stone procedure. Lucky, I guess."

"So it's acute?"

"As in it came on suddenly?" I ask.

"Yes."

"Yeah, but something had to trigger it, right? I mean, it's genetic, but the mutation had to be activated somehow."

"Could be any number of things."

"He'd been working out a lot. Maybe he pushed himself too hard."

Erik stares again, smiling this time. "Jason, exercise did not give your father cancer."

"Damn. I was hoping to use it as an excuse to cancel my gym membership."

He laughs, finally accepting that humor is the only means I have of coping with any of this.

Sledgehammer

Though age has calmed him, so many of my childhood memories of Dad are anchored by his ridiculous, often hilarious outbursts. By the time I was eight or nine, I could see that Dad was less settled and more angst-ridden than my friends' fathers. I understand now that much of this came from his fear of stagnation. The mind-numbing predictability of going to work, coming home, having dinner, going to bed, getting up, going to work, coming home, having dinner, going to bed, getting up.... This is what killed his own father. Avoiding it was the gas in Dad's tank. But he rarely sought out new experiences. Instead, he waited, poised to pounce on any opportunity to demolish his routine and rebuild.

Most fathers respond to restlessness with golf, fishing, skeet shooting, boating, or chest waxing, but Dad didn't care about "man time" or getting away from his family. He desired real challenges, true change, not trifling corrections for a mundane life. In 1986, when I was thirteen, the Syracuse University study-abroad program in Florence, Italy, offered Dad a one-year teaching position. He accepted the offer without hesitation.

Uprooting our lives would be "hard," he said, "but easy isn't good enough."

I disagreed. "Easy is great! And what about my band? We might have a gig at the community pool! We're changing our name from *Bearded Clam* to *Clam*, so it's a real possibility now! And I have friends! And, and, and, umm . . . I know how to work the microwave." Leaving home was not an option for me. I swore I would stay in Delaware while they went to Italy.

Seeing that I'd gone emotionally feral, Dad attempted to tame me by asking for my help with a project. I didn't much care for "projects," but when he told me what it was, I started salivating.

We wouldn't be leaving for six months, and Dad needed a home office in which he could work nights and weekends while preparing to teach new classes in international and Italian politics. Already feeling impulsive, he decided to demolish the old coal room to make an office. And what better way for a thirteen-year-old boy to work through his frustrations than with a sledgehammer, four concrete walls, and the thrilling opportunity to, at any time, turn his new weapon on his father and captor? In retrospect, it was bold of him to include me.

I was already almost six feet tall, but weighed only 130 pounds. Dad gave me the ceremonial first swing. The hammer was heavier than I expected, and I whiffed, lost my balance, and stumbled. Dad didn't make a sound. He stood back—way back—and let me continue until I did some real damage. After the fourth swing, the wall started to show some weakness. An animal sensing vulnerability in its prey, I continued to attack until there was nothing but rubble remaining. *Is there anything else I can destroy?* Dad's edits to the *Father to Son* book suggest he garnered some wisdom from this experience (and the countless others like it).

Lesson: "Hug him before bedtime every night. Even when he's eighteen."

Dad's revision: "Even if he threatens to punch you!"

The four-by-eight-foot space cleared, I helped him with framing, and hammered in some drywall, but eventually grew tired of taking orders and left him to finish the job himself—I presume happily.

When complete, the office was a luxurious solitary confinement cell—exactly what he wanted. Surrounded by thick books with foreign names and tiny type, he would make amends, read the classics, reinvent himself, stop straightening his hair, and change his name to Michael X.

Dad worked tirelessly preparing new lectures and syllabi. The only noises drifting from his cell were those of him banging on the wall to let me know I was playing my drums too loudly. I'd never seen him so committed to anything.

But, of course, a few hours of demolition hadn't convinced me to move to a country shaped like a boot. Mom and Dad sweetened the deal by suggesting I invite a friend to join us. Why take one teenager abroad when you can take two? I knew only one kid in Delaware who craved adventure enough to say yes.

Sigmund Polk Jones, or SP, and I had been close childhood friends, but we had grown distant in recent years due to his excessive weirdness. Still, I asked SP, and he accepted our offer. It was odd for a thirteen-year-old to up and leave for Europe with his friend's parents, but SP wasn't normal. By the age of twelve, he had thick black leg hair, a man-sized penis, wore colorful neckties to school, and had "dear friends" who were girls.

The trip was an annoying mess before it began, and not simply because Sigmund had already started wearing a beret in anticipation of extreme Euro-ness. After marching through the scanner in the

Columbus airport, the four of us stood waiting as Dad's carry-on bag passed through the X-ray machine. The conveyor belt paused, reversed, and then stopped. The agent motioned for a colleague to come over. They spoke, pointed, and nodded. The belt started again, and when Dad's bag appeared, he reached for it, but the grizzlier of the two agents plucked it off first.

"Is this your bag, sir?"

"Yes. Yes, it is," Dad answered.

"Do I have your permission to inspect this bag, sir?"

"Do I have a choice?" he asked, unable to resist an opportunity to broach the subject of civil liberties.

He was about to make a scene, so I blurted out, "Oh, yeah right, he totally has a gun in there."

The airport fell silent, except for a snapping noise, which I think came from the ligaments in Dad's neck as he whipped around to disown me with his eyes. Had this occurred after 9/11, we might have missed our international flight while a powdery latex glove attached to a GED recipient searched Dad's cavities.

Two more men came from a back room; one of them requested ID and asked, "Is this your son, sir?"

"Yes, he is my son, Jason. He didn't mea—"

The agent cut him off. "So, why would your son say you have a gun?"

I can't remember what Dad said exactly, but I assume it was some PG-13-rated version of "because he's a fucking moron." They searched his bag and body as I watched in horror. Finding nothing, one of them said, "Tell your son not to joke around like that."

"Oh, don't worry, I will," he responded.

Walking to our gate, Dad was quiet, brooding, and probably regretting every decision he'd made over the last six months. Mom and I were silent; we knew that saying anything might spark an outburst. But SP, the new member in our small family, naïvely muttered, "We're not in Kansas anymore." I imagined running back to the agents for protection, but Dad laughed. Then Mom laughed, and SP joined them, pleased that he'd impressed the grown-ups with his maturity. Sigmund was glad we were leaving "Kansas," and all I could think of was throwing my new brother onto the tarmac.

After landing in Rome, jet-lagged and overburdened with luggage, Dad decided that instead of taking the train to Florence (like sane people might), we'd be better off renting a car. My mother's father had told him it was a breeze. Unlike Dad, my grandfather was calm and affable.

When the attendant saw our mountain of bags, he chuckled and pointed to a white cargo van. Instead of the Fiat Dad envisioned driving, he would have to commandeer a beast three times its size. It was also August, and if you've spent your life thus far avoiding Italy in the late summer, there's no reason to die of heatstroke now. It was easily a hundred degrees and the van had no air-conditioning, because sweat is sexy on Italians.

By the time our van was cruising down the autostrade with taxis and cars whizzing by us and honking, Dad's shoulders were soaking wet. I remember Mom looking over in support, but Dad waved her off, beads of sweat flying from his wrist. I glanced at SP sitting next to me. We were both a little frightened, but I was happy not to be alone.

Dad might have been able to handle this stress by himself, but with so much human luggage, I'm sure he was pretty jacked-up on that paternal cocktail of angst, no doubt thinking, "Jesus, not only is Jody here, but also Jason and this other kid in the backseat dressed like a poet. What the fuck have I done?"

For the first time in decades he probably prayed, prayed to return to the mind-numbing routine of his old life.

If he did, it didn't work.

Soon after exiting the autostrade, Dad made a wrong turn, placing us in Florence's medieval center. Built when humans still had furry feet and died before the age of thirty, its cobblestone streets are barely large enough to accommodate one obese American, much less a cargo van. We were probably visible from space, a giant white dot ticking through terra-cotta roofs and domed cathedrals.

Dad reached out to pull back the van's side mirror as a friendly Italian guided us through the archway where Dante met Beatrice. "There's no fucking way I'm getting through there!" he yelled with little regard for whether he was understood. We were everything Europeans already knew about Americans: big, entitled, and stressed out.

Finally arriving at 90 Via Iacopo Nardi, our new landlord, Signor Fiorvanti met us. He was a small man with a gray goatee and horn-rimmed glasses: Italy's answer to Colonel Sanders. When Dad used what he calls "Sid Caesar Italian" to communicate that we were from the United States, Signor Fiorvanti broke into a broad smile. He let out a hearty chuckle, and in a jowly staccato rumbled, "Chattanooga! Chattanooga! Chattanooga!" Dad laughed nervously. "Yes, Chattanooga. That's in Tennessee."

After napping, we went out to dinner. Northern Italian food has a way of vanquishing regret and anxiety, and feeling satiated (a difficult achievement for a thirteen-year-old), I looked at Dad and asked, "Can we stay two years?" He laughed. Then Mom laughed, and, after seeing that I'd impressed his new parents with my adorable teen wit, SP laughed, too.

It was somewhat of a shock for SP to slide into our one-child family. His home in Delaware was chaotic, with two demanding toddler siblings. I think his parents were relieved that their eldest preferred to be a free agent. Dad was nervous being in charge of two teens in a foreign country, and he frequently clashed with SP.

One afternoon, a few months into our stay, Sigmund and I were lying on our twin beds having what we thought was a deep discussion about U2's *The Unforgettable Fire*. Dad burst in. He was waving two sheets of paper, and I knew somebody was in deep shit, but I was relieved to find out it wasn't me.

Throwing the papers at Sigmund, Dad screamed, "If you're going to write letters to your friends calling me an asshole, you shouldn't leave them lying around for anyone to read." He stormed out, and SP started crying and ran out of the room, chasing him to apologize. I stayed in bed, smiled, and continued listening to the track "Pride (In the Name of Love)." For the first time in my life, I saw Dad fathering another kid, and I liked it. I wasn't the sole source of Dad's stress. Apparently, it could grow anywhere if properly seeded.

Soon thereafter, Sigmund ditched the beret. He continued to wear wacky ties, dress shirts, colorful shoes, and sport coats with the sleeves rolled up. I pretended not to know him until I saw how popular he was. The other students at the American School of Florence—a mix of wealthy bilingual Italians, American military brats, and expat kids—

loved SP's Phil Collins look, especially his new girlfriend, Jessica, a six-foot-tall Dutch girl rumored to be of royal descent.

Sigmund wasn't letting Dad get in the way of seizing his European dream, but he wasn't the only one experiencing rampant social success. I'd been busy mastering life, too. Via divine adolescent intervention, I realized that instead of taking showers or baths, I could wash my hair in the bidet each morning and no one would be the wiser.

Soon thereafter, a large wart developed on the palm of my hand, which I made a habit of attempting to remove nightly with fingernail clippers. I'd also started chanting "chick woot" like a water-damaged robot. It was a reaction to stress, or hormonal changes, one for which modern parents might seek an evaluation, but instead, Dad just rolled his eyes. "Jesus Christ, Jason. Look around you. Do you see anyone else chanting 'chick woot'?" He might have been embarrassed, but the laughs he got from ridiculing me were worth it. Not only was this trip a new beginning for me, and for SP, it was also one for Dad.

SP never stopped being eccentric. After high school, he enrolled at Reed College, which led to some graduate work at Yale Divinity School, where he dropped out after a year to practice Chinese medicine. I hear he now works at a holistic healing center, the kind my uncle Paul might visit. I missed my twenty-year high school reunion, but was told that SP drank a large, ornate bottle of boutique Belgian ale, and then tried to convince everyone they should put magnets in their shoes to "balance their energies." I would email him for help with Dad's condition, but I worry that magnets would cause all those leukemic cells to coalesce into a massive jiggling glob of cellular dysfunction.

At the end of the year, we moved back to Delaware as planned, and SP returned to his family. But I could tell Dad and Mom were anxious to return to "Firenze." Dad complained about the coffee and that Italy didn't export its best wines. "It's impossible to get a decent bottle of Barolo in this damn country." They started making their own pasta. Dozens of cans of Italian tomatoes were stacked in the pantry (and in the dining room for everyone to see). Dad bought a special antenna so he could watch Rai Uno (an Italian network). "No American networks report actual news," he said. If not for our Midwestern accents, terrible hair, and pale skin, one might have assumed we were recent immigrants. The year I graduated high school, Dad was offered the director position of the Syracuse program in Florence. He accepted, and together, he and Mom realized their expat destiny.

Having overestimated the value of a 2.7 GPA and SAT score of 990, I decided to defer admission to Ohio Wesleyan, my safety school, and enroll in both semesters of the Syracuse abroad program. A freshman in a sea of juniors, I learned to speak Italian, find religious iconography in medieval paintings, and to drink Chianti straight from the jug.

Mom and Dad spent five years in Florence. Eventually, though, as he always did, Dad became restless. Luckily, John Cabot University in Rome recruited him to be their president. Change had come to him once again without him seeking it. They found an apartment in Rome's Trastevere section among the junkies and transvestites. Dad loved the grittiness of it. Mom not so much. After a few years, he grew tired of the bureaucracy and the "bullshit fundraising" required of the job. When a gang of gypsy children robbed their graffiti-covered apartment building in the middle of the night, it was time to move on.

After three years as president of John Cabot, Dad started looking for a new position stateside. It was the first time in thirty years that he'd actually applied for a job. A year later, he and Mom landed in the Bay Area when Dad became the new dean of liberal arts at California State, Hayward. He made good money, and Mom had a job in student services, but they couldn't afford San Francisco, which was probably for the best. Having not driven for over a decade, the commute would have sent Dad to a mental institution within months. The culture shock was immense. It's hard to imagine two places more different than Rome and San Leandro, California—the former as old as civilization itself, and the later sprouting up sometime around the release of Van Halen's first album.

After his third year as dean, Dad realized he was a bureaucrat once again and started self-medicating with single malt scotch and obscure mystery series on the BBC. He exercised a clause in his contract that allowed him to be a tenured faculty member in the political science department. He seemed to enjoy being in the classroom, but he and Mom were never able to find their groove socially. Perhaps after living the exciting expat life in Italy, their standards were too high. The Bay Area is known for its political correctness, and Dad's sense of humor has always been racy and caustic. "Aren't there any cool people in your department at Cal State?" I asked. He rolled his eyes. "There's one guy who thinks he's a hobbit. Should I be friends with him? Is that what you're suggesting?"

Dad engineered his teaching schedule so that he would have to go to the university only one day a week, and he spent much of his free time helping accredit an American university in Hanoi, Vietnam. He traveled there a few times, and despite loving the food, and subsequently introducing the rest of us to bizarre fish soups, the project lost its funding. After that, Dad stagnated, and became mired in the "I guess this is what I'm going to do for the rest of my life" mindset. He feigned contentment, but he was just waiting for a new opportunity to demolish and rebuild, as he always had in the past.

Romanian Gymnasts

After spending three weeks at home researching, taking my pulse, sleeping restlessly, ignoring my own family, and trying to imagine what was in store for all of us, I returned to San Leandro, this time without Lindsay and the boys. I'd become bitter at home, my patience short and understanding limited. Lindsay suspected there might be another explanation besides sadness and fear. She did some research and, much to her satisfaction, found a few sources stating that men have a three-month emotional "cycle." "Maybe you're just perimenopausal," she joked. I agreed, knowing that doing so would excuse my attitude, but I, too, wondered why I was so upset. Everybody's father gets sick and dies.

The flight to Oakland is blissful, a sailing sky spa where the ginger ale flows and the peanuts are free. I get in late and take a short taxi ride to my parents' apartment. Mom opens the door in her nightgown, with Dad behind her clad in boxers and a T-shirt. The shock of Dad being sick has dissipated a bit for all of us. Despite being tired, we feel an obligation to sit together in the living room. It would be weird to simply say hello, exchange hugs, and then immediately go to bed. But after I fill them in on Silas and Arlo, and fix something for Mom on her iPhone, we fall silent. We have a big day ahead of us and need our rest.

––––––––

"Michael?" Mom yells back to the bedroom. She's nervous. We're all nervous—especially Dad. He's getting the poison today.

"What do you think he's doing back there?" I ask. Mom shrugs, not wanting to legitimize Dad's past and future complaints about her dawdling. If this were a normal outing, she might fill the time by disappearing for a few minutes to complete a task on her to-do list: a deft strategy to shift from being the waiter to the waited, as well as an effective means of driving Dad batshit.

"I'm afraid there's going to be traffic," she yells, and then turns to me. "You can drive, right?"

"Yes, of course."

Peering past the fireplace, I see Dad walking toward us, head down, gazing at his Ferragamo shoes. What he'd been doing was putting on a suit.

"Let's go," he says. I think he'd already passed through the frenetic stage of anxiety.

"Well, look who got all dressed up for his first day of chemo?" I joke.

"What can I say? Your mom likes me in a suit."

"You know everyone else will be in sweatpants, right?"

"Then you should fit right in."

"I'm not wearing sweatpants."

"Uh-huh. What's that?"

"It's a sweatshirt," I respond, realizing there's little difference. It's ridiculous for a man in his forties to wear a hoodie and Puma loafers unless he's in the Beastie Boys. None of us knew the proper attire for chemotherapy. There's definitely no dress code for spectators. This is outpatient stuff, anyway. We have plans to go to lunch afterward, and I prefer to be comfortable while eating.

"Do you really think I shouldn't wear this?" Dad asks.

"I think you look nice," Mom says.

"Dapper," I add.

Mom closes the apartment door, locking the handle and both dead bolts. "I usually don't do that last one unless we're leaving town." She has a smudge of red lipstick on her front tooth. I feel a twinge of guilt, like perhaps I'm not respecting the gravity of Dad's situation. I pick through my wallet for a Valium.

"I need you to unlock the door real quick. I forgot something," I say, chewing up the pill.

"Yup, no problem," Mom answers.

Dad rolls his eyes. "Jesus, your mother is incapable of criticizing you."

"Amazing, right?" I slip inside, jog into my room, kick off my stupid sport loafers, and throw my hoodie in the corner. The only button-down shirt I brought lay crumpled in my suitcase: a Western-style plaid with snaps. Hardly dressy, but it's the best I can do. I put on a pair of shoes with laces, feed a belt through the loops of my jeans (I don't own any other pants), tuck in my shirt, and check the mirror. I look like a cowboy spiffed up for happy hour at a hotel bar.

"Nice shirt," Dad says. I know he hates it, but less so than the hoodie.

"You look nice," Mom says as we enter the elevator.

"Thanks."

Dad has always been anxious to complete whatever he's doing. Always worried he'll be late, he usually arrives early. As a kid, I saw him mostly on weekends, and even then he found it difficult to relax unless we had big plans. When I was six or seven, Dad decided one Sunday morning that he and I would go to the Columbus Zoo. Jack Hanna had recently overseen a large renovation. It included wooden bridges overlooking lush tiger habitats, scum-free tanks for marine life, peacocks prancing the grounds, chimpanzees that didn't pace their cages like death-row inmates, and other upgrades that are now expected in modern zoos.

That Sunday morning, I was taking a long time getting dressed, and I'm sure Dad was eager to get going. I had become compulsive about selecting my clothes, insisting on shirts with "stripes on the front, stripes on back, and numbers on the sleeves." Such shirts are rare, and I threw fits when I didn't have a clean one, so Bopie, my maternal grand-mother, began making them for me. Bopie's given name was Roberta, but, consistent with other ridiculous Southern traditions like pie with nuts in it, her Georgia family insisted she have a nickname: Topie. And I had trouble with T sounds. Bopie maintained a thick Southern accent, which I imagine she practiced nightly while petting a large ripe peach. She was a self-taught seamstress with a lot of confidence. The shirts she made had uneven sleeves and strange spots of random color that Dad suspected were subtle nods to the Confederacy: a small blue X hidden in a stripe, a red star between the numbers on back. I think it was more likely that Bopie spilled some of her favorite drink, Irish Mist, or pricked her finger while working. She had shaky hands and poor eyesight.

It was only a thirty-minute drive to the zoo, but in those pre-air-conditioning and pre–DVD player days, thirty minutes was the modern equivalent of five hours for a parent. Luckily, the lack of seatbelt laws allowed me to lounge inside a pillow fort in the way-way-back of the station wagon. Sometimes I would climb up front to stand next to Dad as he yelled at the "morons" on talk radio.

He was probably wondering what the hell could take a kid so long to choose between four identical shirts. But he managed not to rush me. On special occasions he was calm, steady, and happy, like he is now with his grandsons. His patience paid off. When I came downstairs, I was wearing the outfit Mom bought me for my uncle's wedding the year prior: a white dress shirt and a tiny brown clip-on bow tie. The shirt was a little too small, but I still managed to tuck it into my high-water jeans. Dad took a picture. He was proud to be escorting Alfalfa to the zoo.

———

On our way to the appointment, Dad's suit coat hangs in the backseat, flapping against Mom's head.

"Isn't that bugging you?" I ask.

"What? Oh, I didn't even notice," she responds, as the coat shifts during a turn to cover nearly half her face. She's too nervous to change anything.

"Jody, you can move my damn jacket if you want."

Mom pins it to the window with her hand, "No, no. It's fine."

"Okay, then." He looks at me and rolls his eyes. It's the only moment we share during the twenty-minute drive to the hospital. Aside from Dad questioning the navigation system, as well as the two other GPS devices he insists on using as backup, none of us speaks much at all. I assume we have the same thing on our minds. Or maybe my aggressive East Coast driving has them paralyzed with fear.

When the elevator doors open, I am reminded that all hospital waiting rooms look the same. The chairs are purple and barely comfortable: cheap without being utilitarian. The carpet is thin with a dense floral pattern to hide stains (urine, blood, lattes, and so on). The tables are made of dark laminated wood and smattered with wellness magazines and pamphlets outlining the treatment options for diseases to which I thought my family was immune. An acoustic rendition of "Sailing" by Christopher Cross plays on a loop, but not quite loudly enough to determine if it is indeed "Sailing" by Christopher Cross.

Dad has been here before. It's the same building where, just a few weeks ago, the doctor said his options were to start chemotherapy immediately or check himself into hospice and die within three months. The doctor recanted later, in favor of a softer diagnosis, but I'm sure Dad's still rattled from it.

The three of us sit in silence, messing with our phones. For the first time, this all feels real. In a few hours, Dad's blood will be filled with some toxic garbage that we hope might reteach his bone marrow how to make functioning blood cells again. It seems like magic, but what other choice do we have?

I notice a short-haired woman rush up to the reception desk. She's panting. "I'm mother fuckin' late because some goddamn Korean lady was walkin' slow as shit," she tells the receptionist, who stares at her while sipping the last drops of the soda from her McDonald's Extra Value Meal.

"When was your appointment, ma'am?"

"Two-thirty," she answers, scanning the room to see if anyone else is paying attention.

Tragically, she catches my eye.

"I'm late for my damn chemotherapy for the second time this month!"

I smile. "Well, I'm sure they can still fit you in."

Dad looks up. "What? Who are you talking to?"

Now he's on the hook, too. "Whatchu here fo'?" she asks him. "The chemotherapy?"

"Yes, I'm here for my first round of chemotherapy," Dad answers professionally, hoping it might discourage any further discussion.

"Ma'am?" says the receptionist. "Your appointment was for two PM."

"Yeah, *I know that*. What I'm tellin' you is that I'm late for that appointment because a Korean lady was takin' her sweet time in the hallway and then in the elevator she up and pressed the wrong damn button and now we all in the basement and I'm thinkin', shit, I'm gonna be late for my chemo again. Second time this month!"

She turns back to Dad. "What kind of cancer you got? Mine's in the colon."

"Oh, umm, I'm being treated for leukemia."

Uninterested in his answer, she continues, "I shouldn't get so upset about all this. It's bad for my colon and all, but damn that woman was walkin' slow. You ever get behind a slow-ass Korean lady like that?"

"I believe I have experienced something similar, yes," Dad responds, as I wince. Mom still hasn't looked up from her phone. She's smart like that.

The short-haired lady, no longer panting, showed a little vulnerability. "I got this upset last time I was late and it got my blood pressure all up in the high range."

I see this as an opening to shift the conversation toward an ending. "Life is just too short to get upset about stuff like this, right?"

"Whatchu know about life? I'm seventy-five years old. You wanna know about life? Oh, I been there. I been there and back again! Ain't nobody no how gonna tell me nothing about livin'. Let me tell you . . ."

I interrupt her. "Well, you don't look seventy-five." When I don't know what else to do, I compliment people. She waves me off and turns her attention back to the receptionist, who is still typing. "I can fit you in at three," she says, not making eye contact. The short-haired lady seems pleased. She prances to a chair across the room, sits down, pulls out a compact, and applies some lipstick. I look over at Dad, expecting him to acknowledge how bizarre this all is, but find him stoic.

Mom finally looks up and smiles naïvely. The red smudge of lipstick on her tooth is still there, but faded.

"You've got a thing on your . . . ," I say, motioning to her mouth. She takes out her compact, looks at her teeth, and wipes off the lipstick with her index finger.

A nearby door opens and a head peeks out. "Mr. Good?"

It's our turn.

Before this visit, it had been twenty-two years since the three of us were in a hospital together. In 1989 we rushed to Grady Memorial in Delaware, Ohio, because I was getting a nose job. This was not elective plastic surgery. A fellow classmate gripped a roll of quarters in his fist and shattered my nose with one punch. And I deserved it.

Delaware was a socially and economically divided town. I was smart enough to excel in school, but I opted instead to make fart noises and draw pot leaves on my desk. When the bell rang and school ended, I would hurl insults from the passenger window of a friend's car as we drove around aimlessly. It was cowardly, and I was one of the very best at it, but I didn't always choose the safest targets. I forget the exact heckle I used on Jeff Doolittle, but I imagine it was something about his clothes or hair. Those were my go-to topics. Jeff found me the next day and said something to the tune of "You and me, motherfucker." It was all very *Three O'Clock High*.

The fight was set, and the whole school knew about it. Jason Good vs. Jeff Doolittle: Lincoln Field. A symbolic battle between the haves and the have-nots in which I was the snotty, sheltered villain and my nemesis was the fatherless son of a waitress.

I was taller and had a longer reach. Jeff was physically dense and emotionally worn from beatings he'd received at the hands of his vicious older brother. I had no intention of going through with this fight. Clearly, Jeff would bludgeon me, so when it was time to rumble, I swallowed what little pride I had, apologized, reasoned, and bonded with my foe. The crowd jeered as I shook Jeff's rough, clammy hand. I think he was embarrassed to have backed down from a fight. I, however, was relieved that my heart rate had dipped below two hundred for the first time in hours.

I thought I'd avoided the conflict. Then, in my peripheral vision, I saw someone running toward me. Gary Maynard's long greasy hair followed him like a cape. He was a small man, but a man, nonetheless— a senior of legal drinking age. I ran from him in a zigzag pattern as if fleeing an alligator. Within a minute, Gary succumbed to a coughing fit. "Fuckin' pussy," he yelled, wheezing. I continued to dart about the field until my best friend, Jeremy, caught up to me. "Dude, it's fine. He's gone."

Leaving our school bloodthirsty, Jeremy and I walked back to my house. Mom was sitting on the front porch. "Someone named Jeff stopped by and said he wanted to see you," she said, confused.

"Oh, okay. Cool." I assumed Jeff just wanted to connect with his newest pal. He only lived a couple blocks away, so Jeremy and I walked over. When I knocked on the door, his older brother answered, turned his head back into the house, and yelled, "Hey, pussy! That pussy's here."

Jeff rhino-ed his way through the front door, pushed me down the steps, spun me around, and cold-cocked me. I fell to my knees. Not knowing what happened, only that my face was numb and bloody, I heard Jeff yell, "Your nose is *broke*, motherfucker! You want some more?"

"No, thank you," I answered politely. With that, Jeff stormed back onto the porch, where his brother patted him on the back. A job well done.

In shock himself, Jeremy handed me a bandanna he had tied around his head. I used it to absorb the red fountain of karma that flowed from my nose as we walked back to my house.

Mom was gardening in the front yard. "Oh my God. What happened?" she asked.

When I removed the bandanna, she nearly fainted. My face was a Picasso.

"Michael!" she screamed.

When Dad appeared, I saw no fear on his face, only determination. "Get in the car," he said.

The four of us arrived at the hospital, and after a short intake, we sat down with a police officer.

"I assume you'll be pressing charges?" he asked. "I would encourage you to pursue this as an assault."

"Of course he will," Mom asserted.

"No. That'll only make everything worse. I want this to be over," I insisted.

"I agree," Dad said. "There's no reason to make this kid's life any harder than it already is. Sending him away will only turn him into a criminal."

The officer was reticent, but he didn't press us. Neither did Mom.

Jeremy said he needed a ride home, and since there was a lot of paperwork to be done before a surgeon returned my nose to its proper location between my eyes, Dad agreed to drive him.

As Jeremy told me a few days later, Dad quizzed him on the specifics of the situation: who was involved, why it happened, and most important, what I might have done to cause it.

I spent days recuperating at home with a giant bandage covering my nose and gauze stuffed up my nostrils. Dad and I talked about my injury but never about the incident. I know this sounds very Atticus Finch of him, but maybe he thought these were lessons I had to learn. There are dangerous people in the world, and if you want to stay out of trouble, don't be a dick to them. Try to have empathy for those who have less than you. He knew I understood that it was time to be a grown-up and start taking responsibility for my actions. I didn't, but change is a slow process.

Socioeconomic status, race, creed, sexual preference, none of them matter here in the oncology ward. Everyone is treated the same, exactly as it should be. American hospitals are the best in the world if you're deathly ill with some kind of terminal disease. It helps if that disease is rare, previously eradicated, or exotically named after its origins in an African village. Of course, if your malady doesn't fit into a funded research agenda or qualify as a public health hazard, that same medical establishment is often no better than a Serbian clinic. Luckily, Dad's condition is worthy of the hospital's A-game.

The nurses scurry about in their Reeboks, holding Starbucks cups in one hand and clipboards in the other. The pockets of their floral-printed scrubs overflow with stethoscopes, bandages, tourniquets, and reading glasses. Written on a large whiteboard is each patient's name and assigned nurse. In the morning I imagine this is a tense time for the staff. "I had Constance on Friday, and she spit on me. Betsy, please switch with me." But Betsy refuses. She has a new guy, and new guys are always easy.

It's against hospital policy for more than one family member to accompany a patient, so Betsy gives us a private room. "We don't want anyone to notice and get jealous," she says with a wink. After the typical chitchat and taking of blood pressure, I escape to the bathroom. On the way, I check out the other patients. There are two whom I imagine are professors of philosophy at Berkeley—gaunt and profound-looking as Michel Foucault. Precancer, of course, these guys could have been lumberjacks. The others are a smattering of different ages and ethnicities. Most are alone and looking comfortable with, if not blasé about, their new routines. I'm back at the zoo, and I catch myself gawking.

Inside the bathroom, a sign hangs above the toilet:

CHEMOTHERAPY PATIENTS MUST FLUSH TWICE.
TOXINS REMAIN IN URINE AND FECES FOR 48 HOURS.

Reminded that everyone here is sick enough to require poison, I flush with my foot and use the hand sanitizer on the wall. There are dispensers all over the place in the ward, and I pause to use each one on the way back to Dad's room.

"And look, my son even dressed up for the occasion," he tells Betsy as I walk in.

"Yup, I put on my nice shirt," I add.

Betsy smiles, not quite sure whether to take us seriously yet. "I like the snaps," she says, before fiddling with something on the computer and disappearing.

"Oh, I like her," Mom says.

"Me, too," I agree. "She reminds me of people from Ohio. Just real, like she's not trying to be someone she isn't."

Dad nods. "Yup, that's Oakland for ya."

Betsy walks back in with a few pills in her hand. "Okay, Mr. Good."

"Please. Call me Michael."

"Okay, Michael, I have your cortisone and antinausea medication for you."

"Now what's that for exactly?" Dad asks.

"One's so you don't vomit and, hmmm, I forget what the cortisone is for." She pokes her head out the door. "Nancy, what's the cortisone for?"

"Swelling and appetite," says a voice from behind the wall.

Betsy turns back to us. "Swelling and appetite."

"Well, we don't want problems with either of those!" Mom asserts, all chipper-like.

Betsy hands Dad a plastic cup of water and the two pills. Dad swallows them. "Wow, you know what, Betsy, I've never felt less nauseated in my life."

Betsy is confused, "Oh, it wouldn't be working yet." Then, seeing Dad's wry smile, she laughs. "I like you, Michael. I'm gonna look out for you."

We soon learn that some of the other nurses, well, one other nurse, struggles with our humor, especially the dry stuff, which Dad and I seized every inappropriate opportunity to deliver.

The next day, Dad receives his first blood transfusion. Yesterday's chemo nuked his hemoglobin, leaving him feeling weaker that usual. But now, with the blood of a healthy person coursing through him, he's acting quite vital, and everything that goes along with that.

Our nurse, Amy, looks down at her clipboard. "Hello . . . Mr. Good. How are you feeling?"

I answer for him. "He feels amazing. This blood must be from a fourteen-year-old Romanian gymnast."

Amy is stunned. "Really, you know that?" she asks, head cocked slightly to the side.

Dad jumps in to rescue me. "He's making a joke. He's a comedian. It's like semen donation. You know when you can look in a book and choose who you want the donor to be?"

Amy stares at him, compelling Dad to extrapolate: "He's saying that blood is like semen in that regard, and since I'm feeling a lot better, he's suggesting that the blood is from someone abnormally energetic, like a young Romanian gymnast."

After an awkward pause, Amy manages the kind of forced smile usually reserved for class reunions and DMV transactions. Dad's explanation had been too liberal with its nouns (particularly the wanton use of "semen").

"And that's why you never explain a joke," I said, after Amy floated away in a daze. We never saw her again.

Feeling great, Dad isn't letting this gaffe deter him. "Normal feels a lot better than it used to," he says. With Amy off somewhere trying to erase any memory of us, Susan, the social worker, comes and sits down. It was too quick of a turnaround for Susan's visit to be about Dad and me scaring the young nurses. Her appearance must be part of the routine.

Normally, I'm turned off by someone wearing clogs. I've always experienced them to be the standard footwear of passive-aggressive women. But when I see that Susan's are Danskos, the same brand Lindsay wears, I'm more at ease. Add to that her soft Zen smile, salt-and-pepper hair, and unadorned face, and it's clear: Susan is an ex-hippy. After she and Dad compare the years they were born, what they did instead of going to Woodstock, and the role Howdy Doody played in their childhoods (they are both huge fans), Susan shifts the conversation to the reason she's come.

"So, how are you feeling about your treatment so far?"

"Quite good, actually. Everyone has been very nice."

"I'm glad to hear that." She pauses, and looks each of us in the eye like only mind-workers can. "I think I already know the answer to this, but should anything happen to you while you're here, I need to know if you have last rites requests."

"You mean, do I want a priest?" he asks.

"Yes," she responds.

"No, but I'd take a Marxist economist if you can find one."

Susan laughs. Unlike me, Dad had taken the time to read his audience. "We might be able to work that out for you," she replies.

"Really?"

"Probably not. But I'll look into it. I'm always around, and my office is just down the hall. Anything you need."

I can tell she's smitten with Dad. When necessary, he can make a Bill Clinton–level first impression.

"How about a medical marijuana card?" he asks.

"Yes, I'll get a letter from your doctor. It was certainly nice to meet you folks." The sound of Susan's clogs fades away.

"Wow," I say. "*That* was kind of awesome."

Dad smiles. "Yup, that's Oakland for ya."

"Jesus. Would you stop saying that?"

"Sorry, but this is just all so Oakland."

"You just said it again but in a slightly different way."

"He's right, Michael, you did do that," Mom adds.

"Jody, stop being so Oakland."

"How is that Oakland?" I ask.

"It's a joke, Jason."

Too Much?

In 1995, toward the end of our breakup talk, my very-soon-to-be-ex-girlfriend became pensive. She took a deep breath, sighed, and said, "You know, the worst part of all this might be never seeing your dad again." She caught herself and apologized, and though I pretended to be mortified, I had long ago accepted the power of Dad's charisma.

His classes at Ohio Wesleyan were always the most popular on campus. Apparently, Machiavelli is best taught with levity. When I was a kid, maybe ten or twelve years old, I remember students showing up at our house simply wanting to hang out. "Dude, your dad is awesome. What's it like to live in the same house as Dr. Good?" I shrugged and smiled. I had mixed feelings about his popularity. I enjoyed the residual attention, but I wasn't quite sure what all the fuss was about. Dad wasn't kid-funny. It took a certain amount of maturity and worldliness to get him.

Halfway through Dad's first year as director of the Syracuse University study-abroad program in Florence, the first Gulf War began. A group of Italian radicals (with whom I suspect Dad secretly empathized) spray-painted "Yankees GO HOME" on the wall of the old villa that housed our classrooms. The students were nervous, and at the urging of their parents, a few of them did go home. Dad had to address the situation, and he did so epically.

A staff member posted a flyer in the mailroom (a popular meeting place for students eager to receive letters from their sweethearts). "Director Good will be addressing students in Room 100 at 2 PM. Attendance is mandatory." Because of his sense of humor and rapport with students, Dad had become a surrogate parent, a godfather, to most of the kids. When people discovered I was his son, I became popular, too.

I stood in the back with my friends Doug, Rob, and Todd. Just prior, I think we'd been drinking Chianti straight from the jug. Dad walked in and launched into a story.

"Two years ago, I had a student at Ohio Wesleyan named Brian, whom I was quite fond of. Brian asked me whether I thought he should go abroad, and having taught here myself for a year in 1986, I recommended he attend this program. The director, my predecessor, was a friend, and I felt confident that Brian would enjoy himself and reap the same benefits most of you have. After a successful semester here in Firenze"—Dad struggled to collect himself—"Brian flew home on Pan Am Flight 103, which blew up over Lockerbie, Scotland." Dad's voice was trembling but full of resolve. "I only tell you this so that you might believe me when I say that I'm fully committed to making sure all of you are safe."

Dad's words soothed those who needed to hear them. Some were moved to tears. A few minutes later, Doug, Rob, Todd, and I, along with a few others, sat in the mailroom smoking cigarettes (this was Italy, after all). Dad came in, and we all immediately fell silent.

He looked at us, took in our body language and our eager, nervous faces, paused for a second, and asked, "Too much?"

We erupted in the kind of laughter that only comes from relief. No one could control a room like Dad.

Aside from two years in Italy, the rest of my childhood was spent riding my bike to Dairy Queen to stand in line behind kids wearing Iron Maiden T-shirts that smelled like dirty towels. We didn't have a lavish jet-set lifestyle. There was no "summering" in one part of the world and "wintering" in another.

As high school kids often do in boring small towns, my friends and I invented ridiculous games that, had we not been somehow blessed, would have led to our deaths or imprisonment. After school one afternoon, Jeremy and I were driving around town in his mother's Mercury Topaz, throwing tennis balls at cars. More precisely, Jeremy was driving, and I was throwing tennis balls at oncoming cars.

The goal was to hit the windshield of another vehicle. Success might have resulted in an involuntary manslaughter conviction, but the complicated physics of throwing at a moving target from a moving vehicle proved difficult. That's not to say I failed. When I finally nailed a minivan, Jeremy and I let out an excited but terrified "Oh shit" and watched in the rearview mirror as the driver pulled over to write down our license plate.

When Jeremy dropped me off at my house a few hours later, Dad was sitting on the sofa waiting for me.

"What?" I asked defensively.

"Throwing tennis balls at cars?"

"Huh?" This was my response to any question from my parents during that year (and the five surrounding it). I walked into the kitchen to drink whole milk straight from the plastic jug and microwave a few Smok-Y Links.

Instead of following me, Dad raised his voice. "Jeremy's mom said the police called her because they got numerous complaints about someone throwing tennis balls out of her car. Funny thing is, she swears it wasn't her."

"Yeah, it was me. So what. What's the big deal?" At sixteen, I didn't know it was possible to get in trouble with anyone other than my own parents. I was aware that kids went to juvenile detention, or as they called it, "got sent up," but *their* dads weren't professors.

"Well, I have to take you to the station. They want to talk to you."

"Who?"

"The police."

"Whoa. What? *Why?*"

"Because they want to press charges for reckless endangerment."

I was frozen, standing alone in the kitchen holding a sausage in front of an open refrigerator. I stuffed the rest of it in my mouth and walked back to the living room. Dad could see that I was shaken. Realizing that his tactic had worked, he let me off the hook. "Jace, we're not going to the police station. But please tell me: how is it even remotely possible that you don't know not to throw tennis balls at cars?" My mouth was full. In lieu of answering, I chewed nervously.

"Do I need to tell you every single thing that you're not allowed to throw from a moving car? Okay, Jason. Don't throw tennis balls out of cars. Don't throw rocks out of cars. Don't throw bowling balls out of cars. Don't throw people out of cars. Don't throw cats out of cars. Don't throw anvils out of cars. Don't throw yourself out of a car."

I was swallowing and laughing at the same time. "Okay, I get it. I'm sorry. It was stupid."

"Jesus Christ, boy, I don't know what the hell is wrong with you." He could barely get it out before he started laughing, too.

"So what *can* I throw at cars?" I pondered innocently.

"*Nothing!* DON'T THROW ANYTHING AT CARS!"

"Got it. Okay, so let me get this straight. Can I throw a shoe at a car? You didn't specifically say shoe." Now it was a competition to see which of us could come up with the most bizarre thing not to throw from a car window.

Dad rarely punished me. He saw no need to teach me the difference between right and wrong or that *lying would not be tolerated*. He believed, as we all should, that people are born knowing how to be good, that sensitivity, inclusiveness, and empathy are our default state. If I veered off that path, a simple nudge would be enough to realign me.

Seven years prior, my parents received a letter from the elementary school. Our address was handwritten and even in fourth grade I knew that meant trouble. I had an inkling of what it might be about, but was stunned that any of my classmates would tattle on me for peeing in the sink. As far as I knew, they had all thought it was hilarious. Mom read the letter to Dad and me in a monotone voice that belied judgment. Was she on my side? Did she understand that a sink is nothing more than a urinal, tipped over and mounted on a pedestal? No, I was not so lucky. "Well, I don't know what to do about this," she said. "Jason, what do you think your father and I should do?"

Confused, I responded, "Tell me not to pee in the sink anymore?" That's what any parent gets for asking a nine-year-old to choose his own punishment. *Take me to Chuck E. Cheese? Buy me a dirt bike? I don't know. Just throwing things out there.*

Mom placed the letter on the coffee table and walked out. Apparently, this was Dad's parental territory. He sat down next to me on the floor, our backs resting against the sofa, the letter no more than two feet away.

"You know you shouldn't pee in the sink, right?" he asked, softly.

"Uh-huh."

"So why did you do it?"

"I don't know."

"Did the other boys laugh?"

I brightened a little. "Uh-huh."

"I bet they did."

We were silent for a minute, just sitting there, staring at the letter, observing its contours. Finally, he put his hand on my shoulder. "You know what?" he said. "It is pretty funny."

"What is?" I asked.

"Peeing in the sink."

"Really?"

"Yeah."

I beamed with pride and used the urinal from that point forward.

The *Father to Son* book seems to lack an important lesson, so I'll add it here:

Lesson: "Great dads teach their kids lessons without making them miserable."

Much of my brazen behavior over the subsequent years was a misguided attempt at commanding some positive attention for myself outside of my blood relationship to the charismatic Professor Good. It wasn't until I was in my mid-thirties that I achieved some validation, and I had to pursue stand-up comedy to get it.

In February 2004, I stood at the bar, adjacent to a small showroom.

"Dude, are those your parents in there?" one of the other comics asked. "Your dad looks just like you."

They sat at a table in the front row. Dad had set up a small tripod for his video camera. Next to him, Mom was cold and still had her coat on.

I was in the golden years of my drinking, blissfully unaware that I had a problem: the honeymoon period before a mole starts changing shape. So when I heard the emcee say, "This next guy coming to the stage . . ." I threw back a shot of whiskey, chased it with a few swigs of draft beer, and made my way to the stage. Dad smiled when he caught my eye in the doorway.

This was the first time I'd let them come to a show, and as comedians say, I killed: the best set I'd ever had. Dad was so in awe after the show that I didn't bother telling him I rarely did so well.

Three years earlier, Lindsay enrolled me in a stand-up comedy class. I was dubious, but the $345 was nonrefundable. The teacher had been on *Saturday Night Live* in the eighties, and after spending the subsequent twenty years in and out of rehab, he was clean and looking to make a few bucks. He tossed us into the deep end right away. Though we didn't have anything prepared, each student would get onstage and tell a five-minute personal story, after which the instructor and the students would provide feedback.

After watching Dad rule dinner parties and classrooms, I knew that the best comedy was raw, honest, and self-deprecating.

I made the genius decision to tell these strangers a story about crapping my pants on Valentine's Day. It had been a hit with friends, and I was sure it would work here, too. How could it not?

"You know that situation where you're 90 percent sure you're gonna fart, and 10 percent you might shit? Well, I was about 60/40, and I'm a gamblin' man, so I rolled the dice. And I crapped out."

By the time I got to the part about blaming vanilla crème brûlée for my loss of control, everyone was staring at their shoes, fiddling with their shirts, sipping their waters. Holding the gaze of a failing performer is one of life's highest psychological hurdles. One woman simply stood up and walked out of the room.

My reaction to their discomfort was to add more graphic details as the story progressed, as if somehow giving them more of what they already hated might make them hate me just enough to fall in love.

After a smattering of applause, the instructor leaked an uncomfortable chuckle. "Wow. Jason, let me ask you something. Were you trying to make us laugh or gross us out?"

"Laugh?" This was a rhetorical question, right?

"Well, it didn't work."

Seeking support where there was none, I turned to the other students, most of whom, I later learned, had enrolled in this workshop to become more comfortable with public speaking or to be the funny guy or gal at the office, not to be stand-up comedians.

"What did you guys think?" I asked.

A guy about my age, in a wacky T-shirt, colorful shorts, and orange Chuck Taylors, raised his hand. He was goofy and awkward but not self-consciously so. I imagined he worked "creative" at an ad agency or was perhaps an illustrator for children's books. I'd enjoyed his story about being a bassoon-playing outcast in high school. I was eager for him to be the dissenting yay vote on my tale of incontinence. I smiled at him.

"I was mostly embarrassed for you," he said.

After class, I went to a nearby bar, where I wrote pages and pages of jokes and drank pints and pints of IPA. For the next three years I did everything I could to get onstage.

Dad followed along closely as my comedy career progressed, and then stalled. I quit drinking in 2006 when Lindsay was pregnant with Silas. She had started sleeping in the guest room because my boozy breath made her nauseated. It didn't take long for me to realize that most of what I liked about stand-up was getting drunk to do it. I kept performing, but without a buzz, yelling at strangers about my incredulity over the existence of overweight vegans lost its zing. Shortly after Silas was born, I made an appearance on *Comedy Central* and started doing road gigs in places like Detroit, San Antonio, and other depressing cities that one must be whiskey-drunk to tolerate.

With a baby, a sleep-deprived wife, and a daytime tech job at the *New York Times*, I couldn't stay out until midnight, much less leave for five days to hurl stale jokes at drunk accountants (the Valentine's Day bit had become my big closer). I still performed occasionally, but I wasn't writing much new material. I'd peaked and lost my drive. I was bored and restless. All this time I'd been trying to be a comedian instead of being myself. I'd used booze to anesthetize the nerves, and I wasn't sure who I was onstage without it. In my mind, it was simply too late, and too hard, to start over. In need of a new creative outlet, I started writing for various online publications (and later print). I found that the writing life was a better match for my dry lifestyle.

Dad wanted to come watch me whenever he and Mom were in town. He knew my show schedule and would put on his Ferragamos and suit coat in anticipation of a night out, but I increasingly discouraged him from coming. I didn't want him to see how disinterested I'd become in something he felt so proud of me for doing. I also knew his enthusiasm about it would annoy me. Had I known how little time we had left together, and that comedy was an integral part of our confluence, I would have demanded that he tag along. But without selfishness, how does one accumulate regrets? And without regret, where would psychiatrists find work?

———

Still in the hospital, Mom, Dad, and I sit alone and gaze at the metal skeleton on wheels that rather casually—politely, even—holds a clear plastic bag half-full of a fluid that drips through a tube and into the big vein in the middle of Dad's right hand.

"Are you doing any comedy while you're here?" he asks.

"No. Don't really feel like it." I should probably try to do a show, so we could share a night out, but I haven't performed in over three months. Receiving chemotherapy and watching his only son bomb his ass off might be a bit much for Dad in one day.

"Have you quit or are you taking a break?" he asks.

"I don't really know. I guess I'm waiting until I want to do it again."

"It's not something anyone should do if he doesn't want to," Mom adds. She's never understood how I can get in front of a room full of strangers and make them laugh. I've never quite understood it myself, but I do know that I prefer it to speaking with anyone one on one.

"The sex doll bit is your best. Do you still do that one?" Dad asks.

"No, not really."

"I don't think I know that one," Mom says.

"You don't want to know, Jody," Dad says, winking at me.

"I'm mostly doing stuff about the kids and being a dad. But none of it is really that good."

"I see." He trails off, eyes now refocused on the bag. "I miss those little guys so much."

"They're the best little guys ever," Mom adds.

I miss my sons, my wife. I miss liking comedy. I miss my life of six months ago. At the same time, there is something exciting about all this. It's depressing, but different, and I'm a proper consumer, brainwashed to believe that new equals improved. A pang of guilt blooms in my chest. *Holy shit, am I enjoying this? Is that* normal? *Is it okay?* How exactly are people supposed to feel?

Before I can ask myself any more questions, Susan appears with a golden ticket for Dad.

The House Always Wins

After the appointment, the three of us stare at the wet cars as they pull into the parking garage.

"It wasn't supposed to rain at all this week. What a bummer," Mom says. She avoids getting wet as if her skin were made of suede.

We had arrived at Oakland Medical Center during rush hour (a terrible but accurate way to describe hospital traffic), so we had to park in the uncovered section on top. Our handicap placard was useless here. The coveted blue spaces are all occupied by Ford Escorts and those ridiculous Toyota Scions. Has anyone considered that it's these makes and models that are causing people to go lame?

"Well, Jody, did you bring an umbrella?" Dad asks, annoyed that Mom let herself be inconvenienced.

"Yes, but I don't have it with me."

"So you didn't bring one, then."

"I'll go get the car and bring it around," I offer.

"Oh, that would be fantastic!" Mom says.

"Are you sure? Because we would really like that," Dad adds.

Terrified of being a burden, my parents always assume I have something critically important to do, like tend to a fire in my hair, before I can address their needs. I'm an only child—both the baby and the eldest. There's no venture-capitalist sister living in Palo Alto who can sweep in to the rescue. Responsibility rests precariously on my sloping shoulders.

I want to yell, "Of course, I'll get the car. Dad has cancer!" I would fetch it regardless, but now I actually want to. I am also eager to get going. The golden ticket Susan delivered was a letter approving the use of medicinal marijuana, and though I haven't smoked pot in over a decade, I have a decent buzz going off the idea of visiting some mysterious, quasi-legal mecca for stoners.

Walking to the car, I try to locate the nearest dispensary on my phone, only to discover that people in this line of work aren't all that committed to search-engine optimization. When I look up, I see it: the dusty tan Plymouth with flat tires. "Dead man's car," I'd named it that morning. It made sense to me: you're only feeling slightly ill, so you drive yourself to the hospital, but then something goes wrong, and you die. It could take the staff days to sort out the whole "Did he have a car?" situation.

After spending a couple minutes trying to load weedmaps.com, I give up, stash my phone, and drive down the squeaky garage ramps to pick up Mom and Dad. I feel guilty about leaving them waiting and huffing all that exhaust. I also figure my signal will improve when we clear the concrete structure. Due to impulse-control problems I inherited from Dad, I pull over the moment we leave the garage.

"Jace, you can't stop here. It's reserved for a shuttle bus." Nothing makes Dad more nervous than traffic laws.

"Maybe you should turn on the hazards," Mom adds from the backseat.

"Hang on. I'm trying to find one of those weed places."

"Shouldn't we have lunch first?" Mom asks.

"NO!" Dad and I snap. To many people the purchase and use of marijuana hardly registers as humanity's underbelly, but Dad and I were anticipating the adrenaline rush this outing might bring us. We've always explored the subversive together, be it the seedy late-night scene in Vienna or the Internet's "dark web" where, given the proper amount of bitcoin, one can procure anything from heroin to stolen credit card numbers and assassins. This is to be another notch on life's bedpost for us. Maybe one of our last.

After my freshman year of college, I left Mom and Dad in Florence, Italy, and returned stateside to attend Ohio Wesleyan where Dad had taught. As a sophomore, I moved into a dorm with a guy named Pete, who had a life-sized cardboard cutout of Ronald Reagan protecting the foot of his bed. Had it been movie star Ronnie, I might have seen it as kitschy, but there was no mistaking Pete's politics. I had to seek alternate living arrangements.

I found and joined like-minded people in a dilapidated mansion named the Peace and Justice House. The path to its front door was marked by a tall wooden signpost indicating the mileage to various politically charged areas: Tibet (13,137 miles), Pretoria, South Africa (8,425 miles), Washington, DC (445 miles). Our mission statement was "to challenge society's dominant paradigm." It was the epitome of liberal collegiate nonsense.

Two types of students aspired to inhabit the Peace and Justice House. There were those who drank Tibetan tea and quietly dedicated themselves to changing the world. In equal numbers were those who drank cheap beer and bellowed uninformed platitudes about the nature of society and metaphysics (a term I once attempted to define as "something that's, like, more than physics"). Conflict between these two factions usually erupted around midnight when someone's sleep was interrupted by a marijuana- and malt liquor–infused blasting of Bob Seger's "Turn the Page."

Overall, I was having an enormously good time assassinating brain cells with my long-haired Texan roommate, Keith. He had a bong with a big bowl as its base, which we named the Weeble Wobble because it never fell down and because we were impossibly clever.

Mom and Dad had been reluctant to untether me, and rightly so. To lure me back across the Atlantic, they planned a dreamy Christmas vacation in Egypt. While staying in an unaffordable hotel in Cairo, Dad and I ventured down to the casino after Mom fell asleep.

I could tell from his hushed voice that he was out of his element. Having been only to Atlantic City, perhaps he expected the sounds of slot machines, electric wheelchairs, and wheezing. But this was a high-class casino. "Most of these guys are Saudis, and from the look of them, rich ones," he whispered.

There was also a handful of other gamers, whom I imagined were spies or black-sheep European royalty, dressed in suits, long dark dresses, and disguises (wigs, prosthetic faces, and the like). Among them, pecking and sniffing about, were two ridiculously tall, shifty-eyed American tourists. We might have fit in better had I been willing to look anything but self-consciously disheveled.

"Go back up to the room and grab one of my sport coats," Dad said. Normally, I would have protested, but the vaulted ceilings, the tuxedo-wearing dealers, and the stares—oh my God, the stares—made this one of those rare occasions when a liberal college student understands that now is not the time to "challenge society's dominant paradigm."

The jacket provided adequate cover for my "Less Is More" T-shirt, but it was powerless against the long, sparse, pubic-like goatee I'd grown. If Dad was uncomfortable with my appearance, he didn't show it. As I've learned since having kids of my own, parents have a way of enduring their children's worst phases. I think it's called unconditional love, but, wow, can those conditions be harsh.

Dad gave me fifty dollars, which I lost playing a card game I didn't understand and couldn't learn because the gentleman seated next to me was caressing a tall stack of thousand-dollar chips with his monstrous, hairy, bejeweled fingers—fingers that belonged wrapped around the handle of a metallic suitcase containing launch codes. Certain that I was moments from being taken hostage, I walked over to watch Dad's action. Fifty-dollar-minimum blackjack tables have a tendency to break the common man quickly, and he was no exception. "Fuck this place," Dad muttered.

As the elevator doors closed, I reached inside my sport coat and found a five-dollar chip. "We have to play roulette with that," Dad said, looking at his watch. It was now after midnight and technically my parents' twenty-second wedding anniversary.

We wiggled past the other players, placed our chip, and turned back to the elevator in preparation for losing. But a thick Middle Eastern accent sliced through the white noise and announced, "Twenty-two red."

"I'll be damned! Look at that. And our anniversary, no less!" Dad yelled. Then he high-fived me but missed, causing him to make contact with my goatee. He wiped his hand on his coat as the other players grumbled.

After the croupier raked up the other chips, worth thousands and thousands of dollars, he slid a foot-tall stack of red ones toward us. We looked around with excitement but were met with icy stares. We shouldn't have expected any congratulations for winning $175 from people who had just parted with ten times that amount. In our heads, we were both muttering, "But, but, isn't it cool that it's an anniversary and stuff? No? You guys don't care?" More annoying to them was the fact that we immediately cashed out. I think they wanted to see us lose our meager fortune, but $175 would pay for a nice anniversary dinner and, as we would learn twenty years later, plenty of "medicine."

———————

The closest weed place is a mile away and named something predictable like Green Oakland or Medi-Buds. The kind of name that feebly tries to convey legitimacy without obfuscating the fact that it "totes sells weed, bro."

"This is a cool town," I say, before swerving to avoid an unattended shopping cart.

Dad grabs the door handle in a panic but quickly relaxes and smiles. "That's Oakland for ya," he says.

After parking, the three of us—Dad in his slacks and sport coat, me in a T-shirt and goose bumps, and Mom in her yellow slicker—make our way to 94 Weber Street. The weather is clear now, but Mom brings her umbrella anyway, despite blue skies. On foot, we pass an opaque storefront bellowing enough incense to mask the stench of a slaughterhouse.

"Well, shit. There is no number 94. The goddamn place is gone." Dad is frustrated, but recovers upon seeing an elderly woman carrying some leafy greens. "Jesus Christ, look at the pile of bok choy that Asian woman is carrying."

"Neat!" Mom replies, in the same voice she uses with her grand-children.

"I think it might be that place we just passed," I say.

"You mean the Rasta store? That's not the right address, Jason. I'm not going anyplace with the wrong address."

As we pass the "Rasta store" on the way back to the car, a dread-locked man with a hole in his earlobe large enough to harbor an infant slides in front of us.

"Medical marijuana?" he asks, shifty-eyed.

"*Yes*," Dad responds.

The man points to a darkened door and motions for us to join him. I hesitate, finding it unsettling that a dispensary can move around ran-domly like the island on *Lost*.

In a small, beige waiting room, we sit on folding chairs with a few other gentlemen, each of whom is struggling to locate an object in his cargo shorts or parka. In their defense, the weather is unpredictable in Oakland, and one can never have too many pockets. Mom is trying to appear seasoned by commenting on the graffiti, but those efforts are undermined by the way she's clutching her purse. Dad signs a con-tract and asks if I will be permitted to join him inside. The manager seems uncomfortable and tells us that without an additional caregiver document (which he can provide for fifty dollars), I will have to stay in the waiting room. Mom and I brace ourselves: this type of capitalist opportunism triggers Dad's "Red Passenger." That's what I call the tiny consumer rights activist who perches on his shoulder when something unfair happens in the marketplace. "Well, then, we'll take our business elsewhere," Dad says, reaching out for the contract.

The manager pulls it back. "Sorry. It's our property now, but I'll shred it."

Dad gangsters-up and rips off the part of the contract containing his signature, stuffs it in his blazer pocket, and storms out. Mom and I follow, meekly.

———————

Marijuana cards are easy to come by in the Bay Area. Dad could have obtained one at any time by telling a "green doctor" that he was "all out of pot." He was never a big weed smoker, as far as I know, but I'm sure he would have liked to have had some around the apartment if only to exercise his civil rights. Up to now, he had resisted getting a card because, as he put it, "I don't want to be on any kind of list." Dad has always had an irrational fear that the government is watching him. Or maybe he pretends they are because it makes him feel dangerous and subversive like Cesar Chavez.

Two years before, for similar reasons, Dad had refused to drive my car. Later, I overheard him whisper to Mom, "Jody, I will not drive a vehicle with an expired registration. If we get pulled over, they'll impound the car and put us in jail." Apparently, Dad grew up in East Germany.

The next morning he made an announcement. "Okay, you two are taking a whole day to get that car registered. We'll take Silas and Arlo to the zoo."

I protested that we would rather do something a little more glamorous with a day off.

"Well, that's the offer. Take it or leave it," he said.

I laughed. "This is ridiculous. Why does it matter?"

"Because I don't want to end up on any lists."

"What lists?"

"Any goddamn list. I don't want to be on it."

"Who keeps lists?"

"You'd be surprised."

"What do they do with these lists?"

"Well, that's the thing. You don't know what they're gonna do with them." He was getting agitated. "You wanna know what the lists are for, Jason? I'll tell you. They give them to a syndicate that uses them to decide who gets the drug and who gets the placebo. And I want the drug, don't you? *Don't you want the drug?*" He was joking now, but if anyone else heard that kind of rant, we would have had no other option than to send him off to a nice place where he could paint and play euchre with other conspiracy theorists.

Now, after getting "bumped to the front of the big list," as he put it, being a registered marijuana user is hardly a concern, and so the family quest for weed continues.

Sour Monkey

Back in the car, Dad starts barking orders. "Go down to Embarcadero and take a left. I think there's a place there."

"Do we want to get lun—?" Mom starts to ask.

"*No!* Just go," we snap.

Mom maintains a glamorously thin figure by eating what Dad calls "bird food" every couple of hours. "Just enough to make me half full," she says. Dad and I eat twice a day, just enough to fill up on shame and regret.

Greeting us at the entrance of the clinic is a nice young man with the kind of vacant smile that suggests he's on the cusp of going Hare Krishna. When we ask about the caregiver situation, he says that one of us can accompany Dad inside. Mom, suddenly remembering where she'd stowed some almonds and a small baggie of celery, announces that she'll wait for us in the car.

Dad and I walk up the ramp, open the door, and enter a science fiction movie. Natural drugs and spiritual therapies are the only options here. Unlike the lunch-tray-green warehouses of traditional medicine, everything is made of organic materials: the desks, birch; the floors, bamboo. Giant ferns and a trickling Zen fountain adorn the reception area. As sunlight beams in through skylights, I think it wouldn't be at all odd for a Roomba to glide by, pausing briefly to nuzzle at our feet. Though we are the only customers without chain wallets, I know this is a place of wellness and hope. Had the employees been clad in white robes instead of tattoos and concert T-shirts for bands I've never heard of, I might have thought we'd died and gone to Hollywood's version of heaven.

Life moves more slowly here. People are happy, and nothing feels urgent. Customers can not only purchase marijuana in all its glorious forms (edibles, tinctures, sodas, candies), but also take yoga classes, receive Reiki treatments, or simply choose to kick back and rap about mindfulness. Dad's Red Passenger can't breathe in here, and after filling out a form and providing the golden ticket we wander into the main room.

Since Dad is leery of inhaling smoke, our first stop is the vaporizer counter. Vaporizers don't burn the marijuana. They heat it just enough to release THC, which is then inhaled along with a mysterious vapor. As the unmistakable aroma of fresh bud punched me in the face the moment we walked in, I am chomping to visit one of the marijuana stations for a closer look. But Dad is in charge here, and spends ten agonizing minutes talking to the vaporizer guy as I test out hemp lotions and reminisce about my sophomore year of college.

After finishing up his paraphernalia consult, Dad catches up with me in the plant nursery. "The vaporizers are too expensive here," he says. "The guy told me we can get the same thing for cheaper from Big Al's in Berkeley."

"Is that a dude or a store?" I ask.

"A store, I think. I mean, I hope it's a store, right?" He pauses. "Okay, then. Should we buy some grass?"

"*Yes!* But don't call it that."

"Ganja?"

"No, that's worse."

"Kush?"

"I don't even know what that is."

"Thai Stick?"

"Too eighties."

"Funkadelic?"

"Stop."

For a few minutes we forget why we are here. Dad is having a good day. The blood transfusion he received earlier, or "doping," as we are calling it, makes him energetic for days at a time. He sits on a lounge chair in the oncology ward, a soft, worn-out old man. But as the fresh new blood starts flowing through him, he'll begin bouncing his leg, his eyes will open wider, and, occasionally, he'll start complaining about how long it's taking for the nurse to remove his IV.

I find these sudden changes in Dad's temperament to be bittersweet. The tired, needy version of him fosters a deeper intimacy between us. I wonder if they can give him just enough new blood to keep him going, but not enough that he no longer needs me. I like him being a burden.

The previous night, the three of us had been trying to decide what movie to go see. It was between *Django Unchained* and, well, that was it—Dad and I had our hearts set on it.

"The only Tarantino film I like is *Pulp Fiction*," Mom said.

"Have you seen any other ones?" I asked.

"No, I don't think so."

My dad was winded from tying his shoes, "Jace . . . your mom just doesn't like violence."

"But *Pulp Fiction* is insanely violent."

"Yes, but it has John Travolta in it," she answered with an innocent smirk.

"Oh, I get it."

"Hell, I'd watch Jessica Lange . . . ," Dad said, pausing to catch his breath, "slaughter a lamb." A great line tainted by an awkward cadence.

Mom sat down and picked up her book, a clear indication that she wouldn't be joining us. "Do you have your handicap placard?"

The dad I once knew might have felt this question was infantilizing and snapped, "Well, Jody, since I don't need it for anything but driving, I'm gonna guess it's still in the car, where it's always been since the moment we got it." Instead all he mustered was a polite "Yes, it's in the car." In retrospect, we should have seen this as a sign that he wasn't well enough to venture out.

At the theater, after buying a "butter tub" (a term Dad adopted from his hero, David Letterman), Dad cleaned his seat with sanitizing wipes. He had a low white-blood-cell count and knew theater seats were home to more nastiness than airport lavatories. Of course, eating a butter tub wasn't helping him either, but it was nice to see he still had his priorities in order. It's important to continue enjoying life's unhealthy pleasures.

With the popcorn placed perfectly between us, the previews began. After each, I obnoxiously yelled, "Nope!" Dad was embarrassed, but also laughing. My comedic goal has always been to conjure both reactions simultaneously. Toward the beginning of the movie, there's a tense moment when, as viewers, we're unsure if Django will agree to join his co-protagonist on a murderous journey to rid the South of its skinny-tied racists. Though we know he will (for the sake of the movie and all), it was riveting. I glanced at Dad and found him equally engaged, his mouth open, baseball hat shifted a quarter turn to the side.

Then, on the screen, in a dramatic burst of glory, a set of barn doors swung open. Before us were Django and his partner, united, and mounted on matching white steeds. I nearly cheered, but then Jim Croce's "I Got a Name" started playing, and Dad and I burst out laughing instead. If we had been alone, we might have been able to stop, but each time I thought I had myself under control, he'd look at me, and we'd both start up again like two fourteen-year-olds unable to contain ourselves after the chubby kid ripped a three-octave fart in geometry class.

I found it strange that no one else in the theater was laughing. Was the humor in breaking such heavy tension with the sappiest of songs lost on everyone else? Maybe we just had too much of our own tension to release. Of course, we might have been responding to the metaphorical significance of the scene—two men joining forces to fight an evil, seemingly insurmountable foe—but we were too deep in the moment to recognize it.

When the movie ended, Dad stood up too quickly. Light-headed, he grabbed the back of my seat to steady himself. "I shouldn't have put so much butter on that popcorn," he said, trying to remain calm and avoid causing any alarm.

"Do you want to sit for a minute?" I asked.

"No. If I sit down, I won't be able to get up again."

"Do you think you can make it to the car?" I saw fear and vulnerability on his face for the first time. We were in this together.

"Yes, I think so," he said, draping his arm around me. It felt good to support him, but he was steadily releasing more of his weight onto me. At six-foot-four, two hundred pounds, he was not a frail man, and my muscles were accustomed to shouldering only small children. We walked slowly down the stairs as the cleaning crew entered. After slithering through a set of swinging doors and out into the harsh light of the concession area, Dad stopped. "I need to sit down. *Now*," he said. I looked around but didn't see any chairs close by.

"Should we just sit here on the floor?" I asked.

He considered it, but after gazing down at the red-and-gold-checkered carpeting, he said, "No, let's keep going."

We passed the glass box filled with yellow popcorn, and then the small room with video games where a tween was stomping out rhythms on Dance Dance Revolution. A young African American employee flashed a concerned look, but the movie had caused me to experience a flare-up of white guilt, so I just smiled, gave him a thumbs-up, and trudged on.

I want to say that my mind raced through all possible scenarios. Should I call Mom? His doctor? An ambulance? But I was focused only on getting him to the car. His mouth was open, gasping for air. His breath was fetid. A thick string of spit stretched between his top and bottom lip. His hair was disheveled, his jeans too short, and his floppy, old-man ears were full of wax and wily hairs. As his arm trembled on my narrow, quaking shoulders, I saw our reflection in the doors. Hunched over and helpless, Dad was barely a man.

I opened the passenger-side door, and he collapsed into the seat. A sense of calm came over his face. He was exhausted but no longer worried about dying inside a multiplex, which is second only to White Castle on the list of the worst places to die.

Lesson: "Remember, he's watching how you treat your dad."
Dad's revision: "You're goddamn right he is!"

We were quiet on the way home. I felt relieved and proud of both of us. I was physically and emotionally necessary, and he was okay with that. Though unlikely, I hoped that if Dad should ever be cured, this dynamic might endure, however odd it might be for him.

I can only imagine what it's like to have an adult child. The idea of my young boys taking care of me is comical. "Should I put a cheesestick on your cataracts, Daddy?" Sweet, but ineffective. There will come a day, though, when I see them differently. One day they will make me laugh by telling an amazing story or making a witty comment. One day they'll assist me up icy stairs, remind me to take my pills, or convince me that it's not acceptable to wear slippers to the grocery.

It's finally our turn at the weed place, and Kyle, a bearded fella who appears dressed for his night gig in a Foghat cover band, motions for Dad and me to join him at his counter. "So what can I do for you guys?" he asks, waving his arm across the glass case containing at least a dozen different strains of marijuana. It's like we're shopping for engagement rings.

Dad wastes no time getting to the point. "Well, I have a blood cancer, and I want to be happier." I gasp and choke on my own spit, but Kyle doesn't so much as blink. This is routine stuff for him. "Okay, so you want something that's going to make you creative and give you energy?"

"Yes!" Dad responds. "Do you have something like that?"

Kyle nods. "You're gonna want a product that's indica dominant," he says, pointing to one of the buds. "The Sour Monkey is popular."

"Great," Dad says. "How much should I get? Like half a pound?"

"Oh my God," I blurt out with a sarcastic puff. I need Kyle to know that I am at least a little hip to what's going down here.

But Kyle is in the moment, a moment that appears to be happening elsewhere, but a moment nonetheless. "Well, I think you'd probably go with just a few grams unless you're a heavy user," he says.

"Oh, I'm not a heavy user at all," Dad says. "I haven't really smoked any grass since the sixties, if you know what I mean."

I close my eyes before rolling them. I fear Dad's getting close to sharing the story of how he turned back on the road to Woodstock because of traffic.

Then Kyle looks at me and nods his head, cocky, like a bouncer at an exclusive club. Apparently, I can pick out some cannabis, too. I guess once you're in, you're in.

"I don't want anything that's going to make me anxious at all," I tell him. "I'm not even sure I want to be creative." I turn to Dad. "Last time I smoked pot I lost my sensation for pain and bit my fingernails until they bled." Kyle's disinterest is causing us to blabber. He's the therapist who gets his patients to open up by remaining silent. I'm sure if he knew he was having that effect, he would have chosen to talk more.

"Okay, so you want something that's gonna mellow you out?" he asks me. "I'd go with a blend that's more sativa dominant." Kyle motions to another bud. "The Harlequin is good for sinking into the couch and watching a movie. We recommend it for older people who don't have much experience."

"Perfect," I say, embarrassed that my drug of choice is named after romance novels and my sixty-eight-year-old father's after a surly primate. The Sour Monkey comes in a manly Mason jar; the Harlequin in a dainty pouch. I tuck it into my brassiere as we walk out.

We find Mom in the backseat of the car, listening to *All Things Considered* at an inaudible volume. "We got it," Dad says, grunting his way into the passenger seat. "Now we have to go to Big Al's because the vaporizers are overpriced here."

Unalarmed by Dad's sudden fluency in paraphernalia, Mom simply fastens her seatbelt and offers a friendly plea to avoid the freeway.

I haven't been to a head shop in at least twenty years. Admittedly, I'm not even sure if they're called head shops anymore. In college, my friends and I used to go to a place called Waterbeds and Stuff on High Street in Columbus, Ohio. I think drug paraphernalia stores in Ohio were illegal at the time, so this particular establishment chose to smatter the showroom with a few waterbeds and some velvet paintings of cats wearing pirate hats to make themselves appear legit. Though we always went there for the "stuff"—pipes, whip-its, bong extenders, pens that revealed a topless woman when turned upside down, monk figurines that popped an erection when you pressed on their heads—we also frequently bluffed interest in purchasing a waterbed. "Tell me about this particular model. Can I fill it with beer? Will the frame fit through the door of my trailer? Do you think my wife who's also my cousin will like it? Does it come with a free monk statue?" We were such charming assholes.

After exiting the highway and turning onto University Avenue, the aroma of patchouli, Thai food, and liberal self-righteousness lets the three of us know we've entered Berkeley. I pull into a handicap spot across the street from Big Al's and reach for the placard. Dad stops me, "I don't think we should use that. I can walk."

"Oh please," I say. "Just think of it as an apology from the universe for giving you cancer. Really sorry that you're going to die. Would letting you park anywhere you want make it any easier?" From then on, he never let the placard out of his sight.

Giant black speakers with red subwoofers frame the door to Big Al's. They blast reggaeton, and from the look of helplessness on the security guard's face, they've been at it for some time.

"I'll be in the shoe store next door!" Mom says, and disappears, leaving Dad and me to embark on our second subversive experience of the day.

A man, who from his size I can only assume is Big Al, works the front. A wiry Turkish gent with a tattoo of a scorpion on his face mans the booth in back, and Dad marches straight toward him. I hang back to browse all the modern gadgets lining the walls, spotting a case containing electronic cigarettes. I haven't smoked in ten years, but figure since my father has cancer and is currently talking to a man with a scorpion tattoo on his face, not to mention there's a brown paper bag containing two different strains of pot sitting on the front seat of my parents' car, that I, too, might be up for something a little weird.

I ask Big Al for a battery and a pack of cartridges, while checking the back of the store to see if Dad is looking and the front of the store in case Mom walks in. My heart is racing, like I'm fifteen again and shoplifting R.E.M.'s *Murmur* CD from the local record store. The last thing I want is for my parents to worry about me, or more accurately, to tell me I'm an idiot. I sign the credit card slip and walk briskly around the corner. When out of sight, I unwrap the components, screw them together, take a few puffs, nearly faint, throw them in a trash can, and then return a minute later to dig them out. No one in Berkeley finds this behavior remotely odd.

I stuff the cartridges and battery into my jeans pockets and returned to Big Al's, where Dad is finishing up his consultation. They settled on a portable black handheld vaporizer for situations in which, as the Scorpion puts it, "You just need to take a few tugs while driving." Dad's other option, the Volcano, is not only painted to resemble a volcano but comes attached to a giant inflatable bag of some kind. It looks like the steampunk cousin of a dialysis machine.

After Dad pays in cash, because he's still paranoid, we leave to fetch Mom next door, where she's struggling to sort out her shoe options. Finally, she chooses ankle-length red leather boots, which I think will go quite nicely with our new vaporizer and e-cigs.

I drive the speed limit back to San Leandro. The equipment and drugs are all legal, but I still feel as if we're trying to cross the border with a kilo of blow stashed in the engine block.

In the apartment, Dad and I head to the family room—Dad's room. Mom joins us a few minutes later in her comfy evening clothes; a sure sign that she is supportive, or at least curious. I've only seen her sit in this room maybe half a dozen times. It's so cluttered with laptops, cords, routers, and various other electronic boxes that she's always done her best to avoid even peering in. "It's just so full of wires," she complains. And the fifty-inch television is "nothing but a box of strangers yelling at me."

But this isn't just Dad's TV room; it's also his personal nail salon. For reasons I may never understand, Dad maintains an alarmingly tight nail regimen. Upon meeting him, one would never guess he has an emery board and professional-grade clippers stowed in a lacquered, velvet-lined box that he purchased during a trip to Vietnam. I don't know whether he saw that specific box and thought, "Finally! I've found an adequate home for my most prized possessions," or he simply enjoyed the kimonoed geisha on the lid. He has other similar boxes, each housing various supplies: toothpicks and floss in one, Allen wrenches and SD cards in another.

Normally, men who tend so meticulously to their nails have an occupational excuse (guitar player, massage therapist, drag queen, and so on). But Dad's a professor. I'm not suggesting that he isn't manly. He is, but not in a traditionally stoic way. If his father ever used an emery board, it was only to sharpen a fishing lure. Quiet brooding men who tend meticulously to their nails are usually serial killers, but Dad's subtle vulnerability somehow makes his pristine nails less murdery.

Now the TV room/nail salon is a marijuana den, albeit an unusual one. Instead of a Rush poster hanging over the sofa, there's a triptych of pomegranates painted by a family friend. On the large leather otto-man, next to the vaporizer and pot, there is a bottle of eyeglass-cleaning solution, individually packaged multivitamins, and a biography of Karl Marx's wife.

While I hide in the bathroom puffing on my e-cig, Dad finds some instructional videos about how to use his new toy. Made by dudes free-lancing for websites like vapes.com and vape-usa.com, we are worried about their legitimacy, but when I notice one of them wearing an Iron Maiden T-shirt, I assure Dad that the guy is a pro.

Tommy shows us exactly how to adjust the temperature and how long we should "pull on the mouthpiece." Randy, from easyvapedigital .com, displays the proper way to pack the marijuana into the receptacle: "not too tight, but not too loose, neither." And it is Kevin, a.k.a. "The Vapeman," who reminds us to let the mechanism "get properly heated up and stuff" before using it.

With Mom going on a rampant "liking" of Facebook posts on her iPad, Dad and I remove a bit of the Sour Monkey and place it in the grinder. Once we agree that it is "a medium-fine dust," I press the red button to initiate the heating sequence. After about thirty seconds, a red light on the side of the vaporizer turns green, indicating that we can now place the weed in the "chamber."

Mom looks up to mention something about an old friend from Ohio who is retiring and moving to Naples, Florida, while I gawk—my mouth hanging open, as the man from whom I spent the greater part of my teens trying to hide my own marijuana use wraps his lips around the mouthpiece.

Dad inhales deeply and, through a controlled exhale, squeaks, "Now that's some good shit."

I have a theory that when someone uses marijuana after a long hiatus, their age regresses to the last time they got high. Dad is somewhere in the Carter administration.

He looks over and catches me staring at him. "Something wrong?"

"Of course not," I lie.

I remove the Harlequin and place some in the grinder as Dad takes another pull. With the vaporizer already prepped, I remove the gray pot corpse, replace it with mine, and inhale a few times.

Within seconds, I'm feeling intensely uncomfortable. I remember why I stopped smoking pot so many years ago: I become cripplingly self-conscious of my self-consciousness, paranoid about my paranoia. Every move feels calculated and then critiqued by my inner thirteen-year-old girl: *I'm supposed to be laughing and having a good time, right? Okay, I'll pretend like I'm doing that. What does my face look like? Do I look stupid? Oh my God, everyone thinks I'm lame.*

If marijuana is my medicine, then confidence is my illness.

My fight-or-flight instinct in full-on flight mode, I know that a pace-and-pant panic attack would be a buzzkill (I've regressed to Clinton's second term), so I force myself to laugh. Sure enough, I sound like a nervous salesman caught in a lie. The sixty-eight-year-old with leukemia sitting next to me is having a fantastic time: his laughter is sincere, and is interrupted by requests for hilarious snacks. "Jody, grab those wasabi pork chews I bought at the Chinese grocery, will ya?"

I am the overeager rookie, and Dad, the grizzled veteran. He becomes a little annoyed by the kid who can't hold his weed. If only Dad had gotten cancer fifteen years ago, we might have been able to enjoy this together.

Mom glides away in her nightgown, and soon thereafter—too soon, in fact—Dad starts yawning and talking about "bedtime." Though he'd never have admitted it, I'm sure he's disappointed that I haven't been a fun weed buddy. I'm certainly let down by it.

After Dad leaves, I'm a bit more comfortable. My thoughts drift to Lindsay, Silas, and Arlo, and I nearly call home, until I realized it's 1 AM in New Jersey, and I am extremely high. I decide to watch a movie because I'm smart enough to know that staring at my hands will eventually become uncomfortably interesting. Five minutes into a flick about time travel (poor choice), I drop the remote in my lap. I feel around, but it's gone. I'd been sitting on the sofa. How far could it have possibly gone? I get up and wander, looking in places it could only have arrived via flight.

Is it behind the Bill Clinton biography? No, just a random nail file there.

What about inside the shoebox containing ear scratchers and fake Rolex watches Dad bought in China?

It must have fallen behind the sofa. No, only some peanut shells there.

The room is so chaotic that I can't find something I'd dropped in my own lap. When in doubt, blame the room. Never blame the weed.

I go on an organizing frenzy. Mom was right about the wires. I tie up the Ethernet cords, put the vaporizer back in the box, and line up the remaining remotes on the ottoman. I imagine doing this for Mom after Dad is gone. Then I spot the remote resting innocently in the exact spot where I'd been sitting. It will be at least another decade before I smoke, vape, eat, or drink pot again.

Enjoy Every Sandwich

The next afternoon, Dad is watching Law & Order: Criminal Intent *and* filing his nails in the den. He calls this "meditating." Thankfully, we haven't spoken about the prior night, nor will we.

I'd been fiddling with Mom's iPad that morning, and I was unable to resist opening her notes application where, among some banalities, I found the name and number of a crematorium.

I walk into the kitchen where Mom is steaming four pieces of broccoli to accompany her lunch of an avocado sandwich.

"Do you think Dad wants a funeral?" I ask her.

"Oh, I doubt it."

"So, what would we do then?"

"I don't know. Do we have to do anything?"

"Umm, yes."

"We don't know anyone here, and I'm not doing it in Delaware or Dayton."

"Why not Dayton? That's where everyone is, or at least they're all close by. Family, I mean."

"The last two times I went there, it was for my parents' funerals. I don't want the third to be for Dad's."

Dad walks in and gazes in disbelief at Mom's meal. "Jesus, Jody. Squirrels eat more than that. Jace, what do you want for lunch?"

"I'm not hungry."

"I have this leftover roast. I could make you a sandwich," he says, leaning his head into the refrigerator.

"No, thanks. Do you want a funeral?"

"I don't care. You guys can do whatever you want." He places an unidentifiable slab of gray meat on the counter. "I'll be dead. Doesn't really matter to me."

"In high school, there was a nice thing for Emily's mom. It was a celebration of life or something," I offer.

"Yeah, sure, if you want. Jody, do we have any mayonnaise? Never mind, I found it. You sure you don't want a sandwich? This is some good beef. Got it on sale at Costco."

I'm confused by Dad's flippant answer. He gave me specific instructions two decades ago. The summer between my freshman and sophomore years in college, he and I were sitting outdoors at Caffè Rivoire, staring at the Palazzo Vecchio less than two hundred feet away. Italians dress nicely when leaving the house, so I was the only customer wearing cutoff jean shorts and a Bob Marley T-shirt. To complete the nineties liberal arts college student look, I was smoking a Camel Light.

I'd returned stateside to Ohio that summer, rather briefly. For less than a month, in fact. Dad whisked me back to Florence after a wealthy Chicago politician accused my friend and me of stealing thousands of dollars in foreign currency. (We didn't do it.) Dad realized I shouldn't have been couch surfing at friends' houses waiting for the semester to start. He was also getting me out of the country to avoid possible prosecution.

At the café, he wiggled his fingers at me, "Gimme one of those." He didn't smoke, but sometimes tried to if everyone else was. Mismatched pals, we puffed in silence, gazing upon stones that were once walked by Machiavelli and at the fourteenth-century palace in which the Medici decided to have him tortured and exiled. Dad was pensive, and I could sense a lecture coming.

"This is where I want to be forever. Right here in this piazza," he said, exhaling. "You know what to do when the time comes, right?" he asked.

"Yup," I said, relieved that we were talking about his death instead of the missing currency.

"You'll have to figure out a way to get up there. It's closed to the public."

"I bet Elaine or Rab can help me with that."

"Elaine can. Rab is too straight to get involved in anything like that. Plus, he'll probably die before I do." Elaine Ruffalo ran the onsite trips for the Syracuse program, and had unfettered access to almost everything. A spunky redheaded expat, she loved my dad, and Dad loved her.

"It'll have to be at night, obviously," he added.

"Don't want to sprinkle any ashes on unsuspecting tourists."

"It's a lot of ashes, too."

"I know. You think it would just be in a tiny box, but they come in a huge bag."

"Don't worry, I'll lose some weight."

I laughed.

"I'm going to order a scotch," he said. "You want anything?"

"Peroni. I'll climb that castle if I have to."

"I know you will."

"I might have to get drunk first."

"That's fine. Just don't fall off."

In Mom and Dad's apartment, I lean on the kitchen bar, chin resting in my hands. "At the very least, I'm sprinkling your ashes from the Palazzo Vecchio tower," I say.

"I can't believe you remember that." Dad slices the meat. "It's not necessary. I mean, only do it if you want to."

"If you want it, then I want it."

"I'm not going to want anything when I'm dead."

"I understand that. But you can have desires for yourself after you die while you're living," I argue.

He hands me half a sandwich. "That doesn't make any sense."

"You're right, it doesn't. What do you think the rest of your family would want?"

"No idea. Why don't you ask them?"

"You don't want to talk about this?" I ask, taking a bite.

"I'm fine talking about it. I just don't have an opinion."

I nod.

"Good sandwich, right?"

"Amazing."

Lesson: "Help him bury his pet."
Dad's revision: "But not before it's dead."

Train to Wellville

It's obvious to me now that Dad suspected something was wrong a couple years before his diagnosis. We could all see it: he started looking old and frail. Nearly all of us experience a discernible moment when a parent crosses over to being a senior citizen, but with Dad it was striking and sudden. His posture, though never good, became worse. His skin seemed looser, his face sagged. He'd fall asleep midday regardless of what he'd done or where he was sitting. I was always envious of that part.

Approaching forty, I was already finding it difficult to tell whether an ache, stiff joint, or general malaise was part of the normal aging process or a symptom of imminent organ failure. To solve this same riddle for himself, Dad conducted an experiment.

A year before his diagnosis and a week before he and Mom were scheduled to visit New Jersey, I received a large box from UPS, followed by a text message:

Dad
I've been doing yoga and 20 minutes of cardio on the elliptical
three times per week. Find a class for us to take in Maplewood.

And then another:

Dad
Did you get the juicer I sent you?

And then an email:

Jace,

Keeping you in the loop. This is what I "juiced" this morning
(see pic). I have been on a juice diet for three weeks. I have this
or something very much like it every morning before I go to
class or to the gym on days I don't teach. Then I have one light
meal, mostly vegetarian, and maybe a snack of peanuts or a
hard-boiled egg for protein. I have been doing 30–54 minutes
of cardio three or four times a week. This week, I'm gonna go
below 200 pounds. I have lots of energy and feel great.

Attached was a lovely, color-enhanced photo of celery, kale, two
carrots, a lemon, two pears, three apples, and what appeared to be
chard—a meal fit for the zoo's finest chimpanzee.

As he did with most health-related endeavors, Dad used over-
zealousness to thwart any possibility of success. His harried transformation reminded me of an *Intervention* episode in which an opiate
addict erases his dealer's number after finding out his girlfriend is
pregnant. But Dad's addictions were limited to undercooked pork and
Jessica Lange fanporn. Aside from moderate hypertension and a forty-
inch waist, he wasn't in bad shape for a sixty-seven-year-old.

I was pleased to see he'd started taking his health more seriously
(and that this effort didn't include beets), but I also feared the Bay Area
might have gotten the best of him. Had he lost our shared disdain for

New-Agey lifestyles? Since he hadn't yet gone gluten-free, or taken up with a free-spirited mistress dressed in Chico's fall collection, I gave him the benefit of the doubt, and I unpacked the juicer.

Then the morning after their arrival, Dad begged me to go to the gym with him. When I balked, he threatened me.

"Maybe I'll just go jogging, then. Did you know . . ."

I cut in to finish the story I'd heard dozens of times: ". . . when you were at Ohio Wesleyan you used to run three miles every morning, and once you felt so good that you ran six instead?"

"Fuck you." He smiled.

"You can't just start jogging again."

"Of course I can. What, are my legs going to break?"

"Possibly, yes. Let's just go to the gym."

I did not envision us in hooded sweatshirts, punching meat in a freezer, racing up the steps of the courthouse, and ending with a triumphant embrace followed by an awkward smile. I knew at the gym, I'd be more chaperone than "workout buddy."

Dad's personality is not that of a typical old person. He watches independent films. He loves Louis CK, and occasionally gets drunk on expensive scotch with people he just met. He might act young, but age is age, so I entered sixty-seven into the dashboard of his elliptical machine, which suggested a maximum heart rate of 135 (a number also reachable via operating a can opener). He was excited that the Yankees were on the TVs in front of us, boasting, "Hell, I could do this for nine innings." Thirty seconds later, his heart rate was up to 141. We were both wearing headphones, so I motioned for him to lower the resistance on his machine. He didn't catch on and did a sarcastic hand motion back at me. He lost his balance and nearly fell off.

After composing himself and completing his twenty-minute workout without needing a defibrillator, Dad forgot it was the twenty-first century, and said he wanted to "pump some iron." He was like a giant baby bird: still fragile but hell-bent on flying.

After doing a few bicep curls with eight-pound baby-blue barbells, his thirst for wellness was still unquenched. "So, did you find a yoga class?" he asked. I had, and I agreed to join him, not only to escape the cacophony of my toddler-ruled home, but also to ensure that Dad didn't have a stroke. I chose a class at the gym because, while I generally like yoga, I don't much care for the other people who like it. "Gym yoga," as the diehards refer to it, isn't "real yoga," and real yoga wasn't something my dad and I were interested in. Or so I thought.

We traded our egos for mats, blocks, straps, and blankets and set up next to each other in the back of the room. After positioning everyone cross-legged to "open our hips," the instructor led us through a relaxation exercise aimed at "centering our third eye." I could hear Dad's open-mouthed inhales and long, purse-lipped exhales—the whole room could. I feared he'd watched "The Art of the Tantric Breath," or worse, attended a retreat. Had he also been wearing shoes with individual slots for each toe, or a tight tank top made of recycled bamboo, my entire life would have felt like a lie.

Thankfully, there he was in his elastic-ankled gray sweatpants and XL T-shirt, replete with pit stains and a naked pale gut swaying beneath it. For him, yoga clothes were purchased at Costco, along with a Blu-ray player, an eight-pack of pies, and a bladeless fan. Deeper into the class, I found that each time he grabbed me to maintain his balance, or we inadvertently rubbed arms during a shift in poses, his perspiration, like mine, was the temperature of a raw oyster—our bodies always in a hurry to cool down so as to maximize post-workout TV watching. He was still the hilarious, left-wing radical who raised me, only softened. Grandfatherhood had changed him for the better, and I was beaming with pride, love, and anticipation. He was taking care of himself, but I also knew that this train to Wellville would be packed with stories I could use to embarrass him. Neither of us was aware that Dad's bone marrow was starting to malfunction. After the class, when he said, "I'm feeling great and full of energy," we both believed it.

When we arrived back home, Dad said it was "juicin' time"—the kind that requires a lawnmower engine encased in a missile silo to turn celery, kale, chard, and apples into a briny tonic that one is expected to imbibe without weeping. The fancy Jack LaLanne juicer he'd sent us was the size of a European automobile, and along with the ten bags of fruits and vegetables he'd bought at a questionable farmers' market, the whole shebang took up half our kitchen. If one of the kids wanted toast, he'd have to wait until BooBoo was finished liquefying his horn of plenty.

While pushing the chard, yellow peppers, and God knows what else through the cylinder with an untrimmed stalk of celery, Dad looked over at me in an effort to connect, but I was too busy centering my third eye, trying to psych myself up. The nectar limped, oozed, and plopped into the receptacle, resulting in a quart of algae-colored syrup. Bong water. The executioner's poison. We clinked our glasses: he in earnest, me sarcastically.

I'm usually annoyed when people claim that food gives them energy. It nurtures the guilt I carry around about my excessive midnight Triscuit eating. But I must admit that this stuff infused me with energy. I was hungry minutes later, mostly for crackers, but at least I understood the appeal.

In the year between then and his diagnosis, Dad continued to push himself, but his routine changed. He decided that yoga didn't provide enough cardio (likely just a convenient excuse to stop) and juicing was a pain in the ass (agreed). Of course, he typically followed his juice with a decadent dinner, effectively counteracting any health benefits, anyway. It's the "I jogged for twenty minutes this morning, so I can spend the rest of the day on the sofa" fallacy.

He kept up his gym regimen, though, training regularly with a "giant Tonganese man" at Bally's who was "really kicking his ass."

I imagined Dad, his shoulders hunched, belly rounded, meandering through a sea of soulless Pilates bodies—those 2-percent-body-fat cougars at Bally's trying to look good enough to throw back a few Jager bombs at Applebee's with twenty-four-year-old dudes wearing backward baseball hats. I was also worried that his overenthusiastic trainer might hasten Dad's demise by demanding an excessive number of squats or giving him an overly enthusiastic hug.

After a month with the trainer, Dad had achieved his goal of 199 pounds. But not long thereafter, his health plummeted. "I was having trouble making it through a whole lecture. I figured it was probably anxiety over the kidney stone," he told me. After having some blood work done as part of that kidney-stone procedure, they discovered the leukemia, and Dad promptly bid farewell to his giant friend.

I encouraged Dad to revisit yoga, but his instructor had moved away. Finding a new one was a "hassle," and as he put it, was like "polishing the brass on the *Titanic*."

Beetle Juice

After a week in California, I return home to New Jersey. My first night back, Lindsay and the boys are asleep upstairs, so I make the most of my alone time by browsing Netflix for a few hours. It's after midnight when I finally pick something: a documentary that chronicles a group of sick people who follow a crunchy, soothsaying confidence man to the Amazon rainforest. He promises that somewhere in the jungle there is a cure for their illnesses, as well as a local shaman who can find it.

I expect to see the shaman of my youth—the bowl haircut, a bone in the earlobe, that leaf (or canvas flap) covering his private parts. But apparently, that image is from a bygone era, and I am at best old, and at worst terribly racist. What I see is a young man decked out in NBA garb, drinking Gatorade, and listening to a soccer game with his feet up on an old seventies-style metal desk. I trust he retained all his tribe's ancient wisdom, but it's obfuscated by the sad but comedic irony of how the Western world seeps into indigenous culture. How exactly does an authentic jungle healer come to feel so strongly about the Indiana Pacers? And shouldn't he know better than to pair their jersey with a New York Knicks hat? Even shamans have to pick a side.

Nonetheless, dressed in his confused, yet colorful mix of gold and blue and blue and red, the shaman searches the rainforest for lifesaving ingredients. First, he makes a tincture for the woman with irritable bowel syndrome (IBS): a term so on-the-nose that I imagine a cartoonish, fussy, anthropomorphized bowel. In a battle of illnesses, IBS would likely stand on the sidelines complaining about its weapon.

It is a different cure-seeker who peaks my interest: a man in his midsixties, tall, thin, soft-bellied, and dying of leukemia. Though eager for a chance at beating his illness, he rarely, if ever, leaves the comforts of rural Wisconsin, and he struggles to find his groove in the jungle. Nor are the others settling in easily. Images of the rainforest are picturesque from afar, but the HD video cameras display all too well what it's like to be in one. I can almost feel the humidity and the giant bugs crawling on me. Factoring in the bumpy truck rides, lack of air-conditioning in huts, and hammocks made of banana peels, I decide Dad and I wouldn't last a day. The last thing either of us wants is to feel hot, damp, and itchy.

Sadly, the Wisconsin native dies in one of those hammocks from an embolism. Before that, though, the shaman had some success alleviating the symptoms of his anemia with large quantities of beet juice. I nearly gag watching him drink it from a hollowed-out log. Given that the group had been drinking from plain plastic cups until that point, I find it suspicious that they've switched to some ceremonial mug carved from a brazil nut tree. I figure this was the director's idea. Fearing his film might come off as inauthentic, I imagine him yelling at a miserable, sweaty production assistant, "Hey you, whatever your name is, go find a more jungley cup he can drink that red shit out of!"

Before I doze off, a chill races through me, the kind one might experience after snorting cocaine, only unpleasant.

"Beet juice, beet juice, beet juice," I mumble to myself, sinking into a dream state.

Standing before me is a miniature Michael Keaton, dressed in a dirty pinstripe suit, looking like a homeless illusionist. He flashes me a meth-mouthed smile:

"Hey there, bud!"

"Oh, hi, Beet Juice," I reply glumly.

"Whaaaaaaaat? You ain't happy to see me? You don't like me?"

"Not really, no."

"All's ya have to do is drink me!" He cocks his head and hits me with another brown smile.

"I guess that's true."

"Pleasure doin' bidness wit ya, kid." With that, Beet Juice disappears, and I wake in a cold sweat.

Maybe I'm still high.

A few weeks later, in January, I return to San Leandro to accompany Dad for his monthly chemotherapy treatment. I tell him about the documentary, the shaman, and the juice. Though Dad prefers "adequately funded research conducted by people with medical degrees," he agrees to get a little holistic. "Well, it certainly can't make me any sicker," he says.

Dad's youngest brother, Paul, and his wife, Gayle, are naturalists who entrust their wellness to kinesiologists, chiropractors, naturopaths, and whoever is working the counter at the health food store that day. They mind their chakras, eat tempeh, and evangelize probiotics. Like many people of that ilk, Paul and Gayle are as suspicious of modern medicine as I am of people who believe in ghosts and alien visitations. No doubt, they would approve of our experiment in food-based healing.

"Ok," Dad says, "if we're gonna do this, the only decent place to get vegetables is the Chinese grocery in Hayward. The soil isn't shot to hell in China yet."

I resist the urge to point out that the beets probably aren't imported and that the soil is far worse in China. If they put lead in children's toys, I doubt they're meticulous about vegetables.

Pulling up to the store, I see the produce on display outside, which seems like a rather risky practice. Why would such easily damaged goods be left without any security? We could have simply picked out a few beets, paid, and left, but visits with Dad to rustic food emporiums always involve some browsing. Dad gazes lovingly at the glistening whole roasted pigs and doesn't so much as flinch when a clothesline of lifeless ducks sways inches from his thick gray hair. I believe Dad's excessive love of ethnic meats might be a reaction to Mom's vegetarianism. She hasn't chewed anything with a heartbeat in nearly forty years—long enough for Dad and I to find the idea of her eating a burger absurd, almost surreal.

"Papa, tell me of the last time you saw Mama eat a hamburger."

"Well, son, it was a crisp fall day in nineteen seventy-six. We were at an Orange Julius around the corner from our apartment."

"Papa, did you know this would be her last one? Did she know this would be her final hamburger? Did Mama put mayonnaise on it? Was it juicy? Did the blood run down her hand on first bite?"

"Yes, son, it did. But it is only a dream to me now."

"Thank you, papa. I will carry this memory forever."

Mom's not self-righteous about her diet. It's not motivated by politics, but instead by something far more frustrating to Dad: she simply doesn't like the taste. "How can you not like meat?" he'll ask, seasoning a raw rack of lamb next to Mom's face. Sometimes I wonder if he's a sixty-eight-year-old anti-foodie, but I suspect that his zealotry for strange delicacies from the Far East has more to do with romanticizing the Chinese culture and sending a beacon of camaraderie to its working class.

On our way back to the apartment, with a bouquet of beets and five bags of frozen pork shumai in his lap, Dad seems tense. "We have to stop at Home Depot."

"Really? Why?" I ask.

"We need new water filters for the refrigerator."

I ask if we can do it later, but he becomes agitated. When pressed, he admits to having a disturbing dream the previous night in which the old water filters gave the entire family leukemia.

"Jesus, that's heavy," I say.

"Tell me about it. Can we get the damn filters now?"

"Totally. Let's stop and get a blood test for me, too. I've been pounding that fridge water."

He smiles softly and stares out the window.

Mom is waiting for us at the apartment. She's done some research of her own on this whole beet juice thing and seems excited. Beets are listed as "challenging" in the juicing book, which I should have recognized as a code for "NO!!!" These aren't neat and tidy Martha Stewart beets: they are the filthy, unbathed hippies of root vegetable society. I pull each shrunken mummy head out by its hair and place them one by one on the sink: Thump . . . thump . . . thump.

I can't help but wonder why the hell we're bothering. It's not as if we're going to pull off a *Lorenzo's Oil* miracle here. Dad senses my apprehension. "Nope! You're doing this with me. It was your idea."

"I know, I know. Will you wash them and do all the juicing and cleanup, though?" I ask.

"Yeah, sure." He laughs. "They look like Wookiee balls, don't they? You know, like Chewbacca?"

Mom chimes in from the living room, "Jace, do your Wookiee imitation!"

"Hilarious. You guys are fucking with me now. Just wash the damn things and let's get it over with."

"Do you think it's going to work?" Dad asks. "I mean, did the guy in the movie really have more energy?"

"Yeah, but he drank a ton of it over the course of a few days."

"Oh, okay. So we'll have to get more after this," he says, washing the beets as gently as he might a newborn.

"Are you going to cut all that shit off the top?" I ask.

"Did the shaman cut it off?"

"I don't know. That scene was probably cut due to it being boring as hell. He just appeared with the juice in some log mug."

"Log mug?"

"Mug, glass, cup. Whatever."

"Well, I say we leave it on."

The beets are looking almost presentable, like campers who managed to change their clothes, but couldn't find a shower. I plug in the juicer, and Dad pulls out his pride and joy: a Japanese sushi knife. I don't know anything about knives, but apparently this is a good one, since it comes with its own sleeve. Dad grins, a performer ready to take the stage. "You have to be gentle and use a limp wrist," he says, displaying how to properly sharpen his sacred blade. He slices each beet into four pieces, and as their red juices seep onto the white countertop, the kitchen looks like a fresh murder scene.

He places them one by one in the juicer. It hums and whines as it liquefies each piece, the nectar dripping unceremoniously into a common two-quart plastic measuring cup.

Each beet yields only about six ounces of juice. Such a decrease in mass seems only possible if the beets are filled with air, but I suppose there are plenty of other weird science-y things in the world (pendulums, dry ice, and clumpable cat litter), so the fact that beets shrink to one-tenth their size when liquefied isn't all that surprising. Then just as he did with the thick green syrup two years prior, Dad divides up the portions, eyeballing each glass to make sure they are equal. Mom has since joined us to witness the ritual, and I close my eyes and chug it.

After a gag and a few quick breaths, I open my eyes, and see Dad still drinking, taking slow, deliberate sips. He smiles at me.

"What? You're sipping it?" I say.

"Yup. This is strong stuff, buddy." He points to his glass, "That's two beets right there."

I am suddenly awash in a disconcerting fullness, the kind I imagine one might experience at the climax of a herbal colon cleanse. As my body serves the beets an eviction notice, I pace the kitchen, wondering: Should I assist by purging? Or tough it out in hopes that a lease agreement might be reached?

"Oh boy. Are you okay?" Mom asks.

I can only wave her off and give a meek thumbs-up, my brow and palms damp, lips quivering. *Is this a reaction to the root bomb I fire-hosed into my GI tract? A somatic resurfacing of emotional wounds, maybe?* I decide on garden-variety pre-barf anxiety. I am also slightly embarrassed—if either of us is to expel this juice, it should be the elderly man who'd received chemotherapy treatment that afternoon, not his healthy, middle-aged son. Fifteen years ago, I might have been taking my pulse after mixing Jim Beam with Percocet, but at forty-one years old, that same panic is driven by a fear that I've OD'ed on beets. How California of me.

I sequester myself in the small bathroom adjacent to the kitchen, continuing to pace like a caged animal: one step, turn around, one step, turn around. With few choices and little patience, I kneel at the toilet, hoping that the mere act of subjugation might encourage my body to put a rush on its plans. I try a jump-start, but I can't get my engine to turn over. Something is going to happen, but it is not to be forced.

Eventually, I bid farewell to the toilet, as well as the panic and nausea. A few hours later, though, I return for what I anticipate will be a routine wiz. But, looking in the bowl, I see pink water. Panicked, I look around for witnesses before jogging back to my laptop in the den. I know what Google will tell me: internal bleeding, bladder infection, urethra lesion, dick cancer. Before scanning the search results, I remember an episode of *Antiques Roadshow* in which an appraiser informs the owner of a Navajo blanket that the tribe used beets to achieve the deep reds in their designs. *Right. The beets!* I can only hope that Dad doesn't know this cool science trick. A little fear might prevent him from wanting to return to the Chinese grocery tomorrow for round two.

A New Pope

By March, four months after Dad's diagnosis, I am going to California every six weeks or so. I hate leaving my family in New Jersey, but Lindsay always tried to send me off on a positive note. "Get some rest and try to enjoy yourself," she'd say. Unfortunately, resting only makes me more tired. I regress to a teenager while at Mom and Dad's place: escaping to my room midday in a foggy angst; reappearing only for meals, mandatory outings, or trips to Cigarette Max for peach flavored e-cig cartridges (açaí is the only other flavor, so I went with the less crunchy option). At first fueled by an obsession with the idea of Dad dying, I am now chugging along on unconditional love and melancholy. Dad's illness isn't constantly on my mind, but I know it is in there, under the surface, loosening screws and boring holes in the floorboards. Exercise would help, but I barely have enough energy to give Bozo his daily beating, much less drag myself to the strip mall Bally's and con my way in using Dad's ID. I think I understand the mindset of people who grow so obese that rescue workers have to cut a hole in their house to get them out.

But I'm not shirking all responsibility. I've anointed myself as the family's resident armchair hematologist. Dad gets a blood test every week to determine if he needs a transfusion, and since the results are available online, I refresh my browser with a Pavlovian consistency. When I find his most recent results confusing, I call Dr. Levine. It's daytime, but my room is dark. I'm wearing nothing but boxer shorts.

"I'm assuming you want to know what's going on with your dad's blood counts." I think he knows I'm not dressed.

Feeling self-conscious, I stutter. "Umm, yeah. I think so. I mean, I'm not sure I understand why his . . ."

Dr. Levine interrupts me and launches into a spiel about how cancer works. When he says, "There's this squishy stuff inside our bones called marrow," I can't quite roll my eyes far enough. But I remain silent and wait for him to finish. A man in his underwear has no business rushing anyone.

"Look," he says. "I know it seems bad, but these are all based on samples. Since his total blood count is so low, we might be looking at only fifty cells. The margin of error on this is huge. These are really just ballpark figures."

"Right," I mutter, resisting the urge to ask if he means Wrigley Field or Yankee Stadium.

Dr. Levine continues. "His platelets are up, and frankly I consider that to be an indication that he's responding to treatment. You shouldn't be looking at these results every week. They're unpredictable while he's getting chemo."

"Then why do you make them available?" I say, covering the phone with my hand.

After hanging up, I put on a pair of jeans to make an appearance in the living room. I find Mom playing Scrabble on her iPad, while Dad reads a Lyndon Johnson biography and sips a bottle of Arizona iced tea with a picture of a geisha on it.

"Okay, I just talked to your doctor."

Dad chokes on his drink. "What? When?"

Mom whips her head around.

They've seen the results, too, and are just as confused and concerned as I am. They relax a bit when I relay the news. I hadn't noticed how tense they were until they weren't.

"I don't know how to thank you for doing that," Dad says. "I mean, Jesus Christ, Jason, you called my doctor?"

"What were you going to do? Sit here and stress out until next week?" I respond, feeling a bit snappy. "He's just a human being."

"Yeah, I know."

"It's part of his job to talk to patients. Want me to call him again right now?"

"Jace, please don't."

I pull out my phone, and Dad looks away.

"What's the issue here?" I ask.

"It's just . . . I'm sure he has more important things to do."

"Like what? Research? Are you afraid I'm pulling him away from an important grant proposal?"

"Well, maybe . . ."

"Oh stop it."

"Good for you, Jace," Mom says. "I'm glad you got some answers!"

Just like that, I've accidentally become a hero; a fearless, shirtless, jeans-wearing savior with one-pack abs and the courage to use a telephone. Was it gauche of me to call? Don't people play golf with their doctors? Why is Dad reacting as if I asked Faulkner to check out my blog? I hadn't yet learned that doctors intimidate Dad. He speaks to them in the same obsequious way he does priests. *Oh, hello, Father. It's so very nice to meet you. You do so many wonderful things in the community.* It has always irked me. We should be respectful of nearly all people, but Dad gushes praise in a manner that contradicts everything he's ever told me about his views on religion. It seems unconscious, perhaps programmed into him by thirteen years of Catholic school. Maybe in the presence of clergy, Dad turns back into an altar boy.

In the *Father to Son* book, the section titled "Boys and Spirituality" contains so many edits that it's difficult to read the original text. Dad graded it like a fed-up professor whose students never came to class.

Lesson: "Teach him to pray for his enemies."
Dad's revision: "Teach him to CARE for his enemies."

I have never been a religious person. Dad made sure of that. But with Silas and Arlo, I choose to share my lack of traditional beliefs only when asked.

"Daddy, what's God?" Silas asked not too long ago.

"Hmmm . . . ," I said, looking around to see if Lindsay was available to field this one. She wasn't. "Well, it's the thing that some people believe created the universe, Earth, and people. All things."

"God is a thing?"

"It can be, but most people think it's a person."

"Do you believe in it, or him, or whatever?"

"No! I mean . . . no, I don't."

"Does Mommy?"

"Mommy believes in karma."

"What's karma," he asked.

"You'll have to ask her."

"Does Mimi believe in God?"

"Nope."

"Does BooBoo?" I burst out laughing, and Silas wandered off. Mom and Dad are the most common type of atheists: Catholic-born.

I was raised to be suspect of, and preferably hostile toward, traditional religion. As a kid, though, I knew that my grandparents went to church, and we didn't. I knew that Grandma Good had something called a rosary, which she'd occasionally fondle while watching Phil Donahue, and then later, Oprah. Following Dad's lead, I sat silently with my hands on the table, palms down, as Grandpa Steiner blessed each meal. "In the name of the Father, Son, and the Holy Spirit. Amen," he'd say stoically while touching parts of his head and chest in some pattern I never memorized but frequently mimicked.

I would occasionally stay with either pair of grandparents on weekends while Mom and Dad attended anti-Nixon rallies and wind conventions, or whatever it was hippie socialists did in the late seventies. My grandparents saw these weekends as opportunities to calibrate my faith by taking me to church. When my folks returned—dazed but happy, smelling of body odor (both theirs and that of strangers)— they would ask me if I'd been "dragged to church." My affirmation was always met with a booming "goddammit!" from Dad and a nervous, disappointed face from Mom. Of course, my grandparents might have brought me with them only because they had to: one cannot get a babysitter for a child he or she is already babysitting. Staying home wasn't an option. Missing Sunday mass could reroute a comet toward Earth or spark a resurgence of the bubonic plague.

None of that excuses their decision to baptize me behind my parents' back. And it wasn't only my grandparents: Mom and Dad's best friends baptized me, too. Evidently, any Catholic can perform one of these. It's a little-known fact hidden somewhere in the footnotes of the Bible.

I wasn't one of those troubled teens getting plunged into a pond while fully clothed. I was only two months old my first time. Ron and Noreen Carstens bought Mom and Dad tickets to see John Denver and suspiciously offered to babysit. If I was crying when they left, it was because I knew this was a setup. Ron went to graduate school with Dad, and despite being a Thomas Aquinas scholar and devout Catholic, Ron was a "true intellectual," according to Dad. It didn't hurt that Ron was a hilarious little man with elfish ears who became drunk easily and snorted when he laughed.

When Mom and Dad returned from the show stoned and singing, *"Sunshine on my shoulders makes me happy,"* Ron couldn't wait to share the news. "We baptized Jason for you!" he announced, proudly, as if he'd done them a favor by fixing a squeak in the screen door or shampooing our collie.

Flummoxed, Dad told his mother the story. She listened patiently and responded, "Oh, your father and I did that weeks ago." Mom turned to her parents only to find that they had done me the same favor. Over the span of eight weeks, my tiny soul had been committed to Jesus three times: "In the name of the Carstens, the Goods, and the Steiners. Amen." My very own Holy Trinity. It didn't take.

I figured these kitchen-sink initiations would have driven Dad to picket the Vatican, but Mom says that when told of these baptisms, they laughed. It was a harmless act of well-intentioned zealots, and, in her words, "too absurd to get upset over. All they did was get your head wet."

I imagine Dad saying, "Well, I hope you feel better about Jason's chances of being admitted into heaven. Just don't let him watch football or listen to country music. I don't want him driving a pickup truck when he's older."

Years later, when I was sent home with a Bible from public elementary school, he responded by showing up the next day offering to hand out Humanist (atheist) literature. He wanted to highlight the political and ethical importance of the separation of church and state. The threat was effective.

I suspect Dad's private struggle with religion is a bit sloppier than he would admit. His defiant stance often seems self-conscious. My grandmother was a gentle, sweet person and a seven-time world champion of passive-aggression. As the eldest, Dad felt a responsibility to live up to her standards, but intellectualized his way around having a pedestrian faith.

I've asked Dad if he experienced anything inappropriate during his Catholic school years. He responded, "No, Jason, I was never touched by a priest." He paused. "Well, actually, there was one who used to come around and put his hand down our shirts, but we all liked it."

The GPS is still suctioned to the dashboard, but Mom and Dad don't need it anymore. Dad's voice is less attentive and more acerbic than the synthetic computer voice, but far more entertaining. "Shit, turn left!" isn't in "Samantha's" vocabulary. This is their routine now, and I am only tagging along like I did so many years ago with my grandparents to church.

They know exactly where to find parking, and which elevator attaches to which wing of the hospital. They know that only Krista makes a halfway decent latte at the café, and to avoid the pharmacy line after 1 PM.

As a nurse inserts the IV into Dad's hand, they discuss how her son might get into Stanford despite low SAT scores and a criminal record. "Have him write an essay about his crime. Hell, that's better than good test scores," Dad suggests. The hospital is now full of friends.

Mom is in a cheerful mood, too, and she greets the other nurses as they passed by our station.

"Hi, Liz!"

"Oh, hello, Mrs. Good."

"Hi, Betsy!"

"Hi, Mrs. Good. Where's your coffee today?"

"Ooops, looks like I forgot. I'll go downstairs and get one right now!"

Alone, Dad looks at me and sighs. "You know, I'm a little scared about what will happen when this whole chemo thing ends. It's comforting to be in treatment, to feel like I'm being taken care of."

"Really? I didn't know you had issues with your mother," I reply.

He laughs. "I guess I don't really have a choice here, do I?"

"Nope, you just have to let go, so they can do their thing."

"*That's* what I like about it," he says.

Dad's always tried to be in control. In situations where that was impossible (car repairs, plumbing problems, youth soccer games) he seemed uncomfortable, hovering over the workers and referees, doubtful that they'd performed their services adequately. Now he is experiencing relief by abdicating control and resisting the urge to doubt. He trusts his doctor, and that's good: like religion, medicine works best in believers. Asking questions meekly and accepting answers as gospel, I can see that the hospital is Dad's church, and the social workers, nurses, and doctors its clergy. When I tell Dad my brilliant theory, he scoffs. Eventually, though, he agrees, but with one condition.

"It's a religion based on science that attempts to provide vitality," he says. "Not a faith that promises immortality. It's a similarly contrived, but appropriate, worldview."

A church of science in which a mysterious medicine is God and Dr. Levine is pope. In the oncology ward, Mom and Dad found the sense of community and belonging they have craved since leaving Italy over a decade ago. It's not filled with witty expats and gesticulating Italians. The espresso is bitter, and politics is avoided, but those are true of any religion. Catholicism and medicine both provide hope to those who need it. Of course, when one leaves a church, the congregation is disappointed, whereas in a hospital people want you to go, and sometimes celebrate your departure with balloons and cake.

Zen and Other Side Effects

Before Dad's marrow started firing blanks, he couldn't understand what people meant by living in the moment; now he's baffled by the idea of there being anything but. This new Zen outlook isn't something he achieved, but rather a divine gift, a positive side effect of looming mortality delivered by a revered Jewish man in scrubs.

That's not to say it was a smooth transition. Everyone knows that relapse is an integral part of the recovery process. During my March visit, the Internet service in Mom and Dad's apartment had become atrocious. Fed up with the spinning Netflix wheel, I suggest to Dad that we go on a father-son pilgrimage to Radio Shack, his favorite place on Earth. Oddly, he takes some convincing. He seems tense in the car, and clenches his jaw when we walk in.

"They don't have it," he says.

"Have what?"

"The modem."

"We haven't even looked yet," I say.

I look over to the pockmarked employee, whose nametag reads "Jamie."

"Hi, do you have any Motorola DSL modems that work with AT&T?" I ask.

"All of our modems are in that aisle over there," he says, pointing.

"Okay, thanks."

I ask Dad if he's coming, and he joins me, albeit reluctantly.

"See? Look. They don't have the goddamn modem," he says, aggressively enough to frighten Jamie, who, sensing trouble, puts down his Mountain Dew and walks over. Dad turns his back, feigning interest in the remote-control helicopters on the other side of the aisle. It occurs to me why Dad is so tense. It's the same reason alcoholics avoid going to bars: they're afraid they won't be able to control themselves. Radio Shack has a Communist feel to it that Dad likes. Unadorned, and uncomplicated by too many choices, it's a blue-collar Best Buy. Dad knows the failure of this utopia is one of his anger triggers.

"Having trouble finding what you need?" Jamie asks.

"Yup! You don't have it," Dad says, turning to walk out. Before opening the door, he turns back, "You know who does? Office Depot, and we'll be taking our business there!" I shrug at a very confused Jamie, and then jog off to catch up with Dad.

"You know that kid doesn't give a shit if we go to Office Depot, right?" I ask.

"Well, he should!" Dad snaps back, holding on to the quaint ideal that employees should take pride in their companies, like cashiers at Woolworth's in the 1960s.

This is one of the few times I've seen him lose his temper over the previous couple of months. Overall, he may have unintentionally harnessed *The Power of Now*, but the secret no one tells you is that sometimes "Now" involves your favorite electronics store not having the right equipment. As long as Dad avoids the marketplace, he's damn near Zen.

I have experienced no such transformation. The train to Shambala did not stop in New Jersey. Upon returning home after each visit with Mom and Dad, I was a little less present, my fuse a little shorter. I lay down more and spent too much time staring at my phone. Having subscribed to the power of five minutes from now, I had begun waiting for the current moment to pass in hopes that the next one might be more pleasant. Buddhists make *presence* seem so easy. "Be like water," they say, ignoring that most of us have emotional dams blocking its flow.

Trust your deepest consciousness.

Focus on he who is breathing.

Why can't anyone explain Zen to me without being mystical?

"Zen is the state of not trying to understand." I feel like Phaedrus talking to Socrates.

At no time, however, is it more necessary to employ these practices than when dealing with small children. The personal transformation required by parenthood is gnarled in a paradox, though. We're expected to become more patient and flexible amid the most emotionally cacophonous years of our lives. Only a true Zen master could be like water while a child plays a plastic flute in his ear.

When in a good mood, I can sometimes pull it off: "Hey guys, instead of squirting all the lotion into the toilet, how about we do an experiment to see what happens to cheese when it melts!" But in between my trips to California, good moods were increasingly elusive. More commonly, my reaction was stern and followed by a sigh and a mile-long stare.

The Goods are a tense and fragile bunch. No matter how much we try to relax, via meditation, exercise, pharmaceuticals, booze (or in the case of my grandfather, fishing trips and booze), the yeasty dough of unease continues to churn in our stomachs.

I seem to have passed this gem of a mutation onto my son Silas. As a baby, he was a fleshy ball of fuss. He didn't sleep. He wouldn't nurse. There seemed to be something he wanted that Lindsay and I couldn't provide. When he'd scream for so long that his face turned the color of rhubarb, we'd look at each other in a panic. *What's wrong with him?* In the years since, we've learned that what we assumed was colic, a physical condition, was more likely something psychological. Silas is a first-grader now. He's impatient but empathetic; a first-born people-pleaser with zero patience for people who are hard to please. Of course, I'm the person he wants to please most, and my praise has become even less satiating over the past few months.

Sometime in April, while playing Lego Batman on the Nintendo Wii, Silas berated me for not jumping at the right times, missing valuable coins, and failing to change into a bomb suit so I could blow up a van full of grizzled shipyard mobsters. So, I let him be Batman and relegated myself to the skirt-wearing Robin. What more could he want? But he was still agitated. After falling from a tightrope connecting one bad-guy building to another, he yelled, "You did that on purpose!" and threw down his controller.

"Why would I do that?" I said. "I'm not perfect at video games."

"You did it to make me mad."

"Why would I want you to be mad?" I asked, monotone and defeated. I knew where this was going and didn't have the energy to stop it.

"Because you don't want to play Wii with me!" he yelled, storming to the hallway.

When he returned—sniffling, wiping his tears, and catching his breath—he collapsed in my arms. "I'm sorry, Daddy."

"I'm sorry too, Bud." Instead of moving forward, and crossing the goddamn tightrope, I made a classic parenting mistake: I revisited the issue. "Can you tell me why you got so mad?" I asked, thinking I was being therapeutic.

"Because . . . Ahhhhhhhhh!" And off he went again.

I turned to Lindsay, who had observed the whole thing. "Do you have any idea what this is about?" I asked.

"He senses you aren't present," she answered, a little too eager.

"But I am! I'm playing this game with him. I just fell off some stupid tightrope. It's sort of hard."

"It's not about that."

"Actually, I think it is about that."

"No. He wants to spend quality time with you," she said.

"How is that different from what we're doing now, exactly?"

"It's when both of you are equally enthusiastic about something."

"Well, I'm not really an enthusiastic person."

"Umm, yeah. I know," she said.

I could never seem to get my own dad's attention growing up. His head was always somewhere else. "Dad, Dad, Dad, Dad, Dad," I'd machine gun until he answered.

Finally, he'd bark, "What? Jesus Christ."

"Nothing. Forget it."

"No, what did you want?" he'd ask, with a hint of repentance.

"Nothing."

"Then don't say my name twenty times unless you want something."

"Fine!" Then I'd stomp into the kitchen to watch Mom cook. She always listened to me.

When it comes to their own emotions, kids are all confusion; either they're unable to express how they really feel, or they don't understand how they feel. Kids are like a perpetual sympathy quiz. As parents, we are supposed to supply the right answers. The more I failed these tests, the more Lindsay and I argued.

Later that night, after Silas and I sorted out the tragic tightrope situation, Lindsay seemed fed up with me. "Why can't you be more joyful?" she asked.

Joy. It's such an aggressive term, isn't it?

Joy

jOy

JoY

JOY!!!!

I was already suffering from a mild, twenty-first-century depression before Dad's illness, so this seemed like a particularly bad moment for Lindsay to scatter plot my bliss scores. The truth is, save half a dozen dates with cocaine, I've never felt joyful. Who besides the intoxicated and maniacally naïve experience this?

"Well, maybe I'm less *joyful* than you'd like because my father is dying," I said. I knew she'd ignore this excuse. I'd used it a dozen or more times already, and it had lost its bite.

"Do you enjoy life?" she asked, whittling my patience down to a nub. I admit it was a good question. I wanted to be able to answer with a resounding *yes*, but I wasn't brought up in the kind of home that discusses joy. Any whiff of pop psychology triggers my gag reflex.

"I don't really think about it," I replied. "I just kind of live. It's not as if I have a choice. It's like asking someone if they enjoy breathing."

She stared at me with a mix of concern and confusion: a cat to a candle. I think she wanted to know why I wasn't *acting* like I enjoy life.

As time went on, this became an ongoing source of conflict between us. Some days later, Lindsay said, sadly, "I can't imagine if we were driving in a car that you would ever look out the window and say, 'Wow, look at that tree, isn't it beautiful?' That upsets me." Perhaps she didn't know that I'm not really a tree person, much less one who might force others to endure my appreciation of them. What starts with trees quickly expands to other fauna, and the next thing I know, I'm puttering around my house with a watering can asking my ferns if they're thirsty. At least, that's what I imagine would happen if I pretended that nature infused me with unrelenting wonder and happiness.

In response to these legitimate gripes, I shut down more, hoping to scare her into thinking she'd caused me to fall deeper into my hole. Physically, I acted like a dog after being punished. Emotionally, I was trying to elicit sympathy and guilt rather than admit fault. And, well, maybe that's what dogs do, too. Let's call it vicious manipulation via involuntary pouting. It's what I did as a kid when Dad let out his controlled leaks. They say men seek women who remind them of their mothers, but I married a woman who reminds me of Dad.

I understood that Lindsay was just trying to avoid popping. On an emotional level, she is there for me when I really need her, but day-to-day I was joy poison. She couldn't help but leak a comment whenever I shuffled around in my slippers, slumped down in my chair, or stared off into the distance. Her father had died five years before, so it's not as if she was unsympathetic, though she certainly dealt with it differently:

stoic, strong, and unflinching in her commitment to not letting sorrow throw her off course or become the foundation of her moods. She was sad, but sought ways and reasons to be content and happy in any given moment.

If it were just the two of us, Lindsay could have restrained herself, but she feared that Silas was modeling my depression. "He walks away with his head down like that because he sees you do it. You know that, right?" Why is it that children never mimic behaviors like sleeping past 7 AM on Sunday? Not to invalidate my wife's concern here, but it's only fair to point out that she, like all mothers, has irrational fears when it comes to her children: random gas leaks, concussions after routine falls, and "sensory overload" from playing Monopoly Junior while listening to The Jackson 5.

Of course, I could see how my depression affected my family, but I was addicted to it. I had finally been given a valid excuse to mope, and I made the most of it. I was already losing my Dad, so fuck it, why shouldn't I lose everything else, too? I fantasized about stocking up on e-cigs, renting a Chevy Volt, and driving west until I ran out of batteries (somewhere in Pennsylvania).

Eventually, after five months of drama, Lindsay needed a break— from me, from everything. She'd been on mom duty for too long and wanted to spend a couple of nights in a hotel with her sister. Of course, this was a completely reasonable request. No one deserved some R&R more than she did, so I agreed with a smile. It's what adults do. We mask our childish emotions with a simulacrum of maturity. Sometimes we fail.

The truth is, I was bitter. I didn't want to acknowledge that she had needs, and I was angry that she would have the gall to attend to them. When she texted to ask if she could stay one extra night, Arlo was screaming at me because I couldn't re-create an exact replica of the cardboard fort we'd built the night before. We'd run out of duct tape, so I was assembling a dozen boxes with an adhesive normally used for wrapping Christmas presents. I usually love my "dude time" with the boys. This should have been an opportunity for me to get out of my head.

I didn't respond to Lindsay's text—the honesty and sweet tone of her request pissed me off. "I feel like this is really benefiting me," she wrote. "I'm just now starting to feel a little refreshed!" The desire to hoard attention for myself overcame my ability to be an adult.

She called me, but I let it go to voicemail. Ten minutes later, she called again, and unfortunately, I chose to answer. "You know, you should do this, too," she said. "Get away for a few nights and escape. You can do it anytime you want."

An emotional switch toggled inside me. Though I knew the words coming out of my mouth were unfair, if not cruel, I had lost control. "You're right, I do need a break from my life. But you know what the problem is? I can't escape it. My fucking life comes with me everywhere I go. Even in a hotel room, my father is still dying."

"You don't sound good. I'll just come home. I don't need to stay another night."

"Oh no, you can stay another night. You need to *relax*. I'll just get back to building this fort with Scotch tape for Arlo. He's out of his mind."

"Is he hungry?"

"No. I feed our children. I'm their father, so I know that I'm supposed to feed them."

"Please calm down."

"Oh, and I'm tired of you assuming that I get all of this downtime when I go to California. Do you know what I do there? I drive my dad to doctor's appointments. And I don't have a sister, either. I'm an only child. Do you even know what that's like?"

"I'm coming home."

"No. Come home when you're *fully refreshed*."

She came home.

In the beginning of my father's illness, I thought I was dealing with the situation so well. I made promises. And I felt energized by them. *My dad and I will talk on the phone every day. I'll learn everything there is to know about leukemia. I will not take anything for granted.* I didn't write a letter to myself or pin these mantras on a vision board, and maybe that's where I erred, because six months after Dad's diagnosis, I was worse off than when I started. I was talking to my wife as if I were her teenage son, smoking e-cigs like a junkie robot, and eating sausage every morning like a disco owner in Munich.

Steadily, my energy flagged. The daily phone calls with Dad became weekly; discussions of test results ended in accepted confusion rather than diligent research. I forgot my password for MarrowForums .org. Things hadn't changed nearly as much as I thought. A psychologist told me it was "natural" and "okay" to feel that way. She said her job was to help me feel okay about who I was and to accept how I was behaving. But I wanted her to help me change everything. Later, eventually, I realized those two things aren't mutually exclusive. I was resisting a return to normal, which was something I wasn't yet aware that I wanted.

I Knew I Was Because I Am

If you've never had a fresh, hot, soft pretzel made by a dude in his garage, I'd suggest you start living your life with a little more purpose. In the early eighties, there was a place, a garage, just a few blocks from Grandma and Grandpa Good's house in Dayton, Ohio. I don't know if he made them for fun, to get away from his wife, or this wizard of twisted dough simply had a passion and a gift. The details of his inspiration didn't matter to us. We always left Delaware at 1:30 on Christmas Eve because that got us to those pretzels at 3 PM, when they were scooting off the conveyor belt, hot and ready to eat. One brown grocery bag full cost three bucks, and there was never a line.

My grandparents' house had a trick door but if you knew the timing (twist the knob, put your shoulder into it, and *then* kick the bottom), you were family and not expected to knock. When we would bust in with that brown bag, folded twice at the top to keep the heat in, the house rumbled. "Hot damn! Somebody up and got some pretzels," Uncle Clement would yell, as Grandma hustled to the phone to call Grandpa at the Red Carpet bar. "It's Detta. Tell Eddie the kids are here." Aunt Libby was usually pretty quiet because cursing around Detta made her nervous. Uncle Paul would hang back a little, smiling. I don't think he cared much for the infamous garage pretzels. Once the hoopla subsided, he'd give Mom and Dad a hug and shake my hand. He treated kids like grown-ups, and we loved him for it.

Paul has always marched to the beat of a tuba: slow, deliberate, and without concern for other instruments. His voice is calming, and he speaks in a cadence that belies self-doubt. He does what he wants, when he wants, and how he wants, but he never causes harm to others in the process. Paul, for better or worse, is the closest thing I know to Zen.

He and Gayle live across the street from Dad's other brother, Clement, in the small town of Goose River, Ohio. It's a place lost in time (almost as lost as the idea of living across the street from one's brother). My uncles have addresses, but you wouldn't need them. The houses in Goose River don't have mailboxes. Residents pick up their parcels at the post office, like some kind of modern-day Deadwood. Main Street, the only street in Goose River that isn't any alley, contains more dogs and barefoot teenagers than cars. It's a great town to visit if you want to feel like you're from a dystopic future, or if you want to see what the simple life looks like. The "grid" looms nearby, but one can't see it or feel it in Goose River. And that's exactly why my uncles have never left.

Clement works at a graphic design firm in nearby Dayton: he's a conventional bachelor by Goose River standards. In his spare time he collects pop-culture mementos. On the top shelf of his pantry is an unopened six-pack of Billy Beer (a hard-to-find brew made by Jimmy Carter's hillbilly brother). Upstairs is his baseball-card collection, categorized and kept in pocket-page protectors. He used to attend twenty to thirty Cincinnati Reds games a season, but now devotes himself full time to the Dayton Dragons, a local minor league team. He sends Dad a new baseball hat occasionally, but Mom doesn't think Dad looks good in hats. She'll have to get over that.

In Paul and Gayle's narrow old-frame two-story, which they recently painted electric blue, you might find a banjo or a '60s Gibson acoustic leaning against the door of Gayle's yoga room. Their bookshelves are filled with everything from Kierkegaard to Tom Robbins. Self-educated, they have a deep knowledge of sociology, psychology, philosophy, and Eastern religions. A healthy soup always simmers on the vintage stovetop, and together with incense and aromatic oils, the house smells of counterculture (or as they call it in Goose River, "culture").

Bluegrass music was something Dad's father, Edwin, respected far more than politics or art. He messed around with the harmonica, and if appropriately lubricated, would accompany Paul's banjo or guitar on family holidays. It made everyone happy to see him enjoy something, especially later in his life, when he was disoriented and irrational. I remember seeing Dad tear up during one of these awkward hoedowns. Jealousy and regret mixed with a little love will moisten the eyes of any man.

———————

In May, Dad calls me at home in New Jersey. Since he usually texts, "Is now an OK time to call?" I know he must have important news.

"Dr. Levine said things are looking good," he tells me.

"Great! What does that mean, exactly?"

"Well, *he called me*, so . . ."

"Let's get over this block you have with doctors and telephones. What did he say?"

"He said I'm in remission."

"Whoa, what?" I open a web browser to find out the duration of remission for myelodysplasia, leukemia, preleukemia, or whatever the hell it is that's been slowly killing my father.

"It's unpredictable, though," Dad says.

"Yeah, I just Googled it."

"What did you find?"

"It'll probably last for weeks or months, not years."

"That's what he told me, too. All this really means is that the drug is working."

"Is he going to take you off it?" I ask.

"He didn't say."

"Does this mean you can get a transplant?"

"Well, he said we should start the process."

"Where do I go to get tested?"

"No, you're unlikely to be a match. If I have one, it would be Clement, Libby, or Paul."

"Right." I paused.

"Are you smoking?"

"Just those e-cigs."

"Jace, if I've learned anything from this, it's to not put weird shit into your body."

"I know. I'm just stressed."

"I'm sorry."

"It's not your fault."

"Well, it is, and it isn't."

"How's Mom?" I ask.

"She's at Curves, working out. She never even breaks a sweat."

"I don't think I've ever seen her sweat."

"Me, neither," Dad says, chuckling.

"Okay, I gotta go," I say. "This is good news."

"Yup, get back to it. Talk to you soon."

The cancer machine still hums in Dad's marrow, but the chemo is tossing each bad cell into a brown paper bag. At any time it could become overwhelmed by the output, but I figure that if I am going to let all the low points get me down, I might as well let the high ones do their thing, too. It's been six months since Dad was first diagnosed, and for the first time I'm hopeful. That hasn't translated into joy or a greater appreciation of trees, but still, it's nice to feel different.

A stem cell transplant is the only cure for leukemia. We'd been told Dad was too old for one, but apparently Dr. Levine had reconsidered due to Dad's lack of "co-morbidities." What a terrible word. "Good news, sir, cancer is the only thing about you that's gruesome and macabre. Should you also develop diabetes or heart disease, your body would simply be too grotesque to consider further treatment."

Dad is conflicted and nervous about asking his siblings to get tested. He has to act quickly, though, because a relapse can come at any time.

Jace,

What do you think of this email? Should I retain or delete the last paragraph?

Dad

Sent from my iPad

Dear Guys,

There is a new development in my disease. Dr. Levine wants to begin the very preliminary bone marrow transplant procedure. The first step in this process is to determine whether there is a donor match with a sibling. If you are willing, you will be sent a "kit" from Stanford University Hospital. The process is very simple, it requires that you have a small amount of blood taken. It does NOT require a bone marrow biopsy.

A successful transplant can result in a cure, not just a remission. However, Dr. Levine says that "elderly" patients are less likely to get into the clinical trials. He added that 50 years old is considered elderly.

If this is something that you are willing to do, send me the address to which you want the "kit" to be sent. If there is any financial burden to you, my insurance will take care of it.

Understand I realize how fully this is a significant request on my part and ultimately the possibility of even more involvement. If you want to opt out, I completely respect your decision and nothing will change in the close relationship we have always enjoyed.

Love,

Mick

"It's perfect," I respond. "Though I don't much like the idea that I'll be 'elderly' in nine years."

"Yeah, how do you think I feel? Apparently, I've been near death for almost twenty."

"You've made it farther than you should have, then. The email is really good. You should send it."

"Okay, I'll send it out now."

Maybe as an only child I have an inflated sense of siblinghood, but how could anyone deny this request? If I received a similar plea from a "Nigerian prince," I'd at least take some time to consider it.

Communication is unfamiliar territory for Dad, Clement, Libby, and Paul. They'd always spoken to each other through my grandma, Detta. If Libby wanted Paul to know something, she told Detta, who would pass it along. It was convenient and effective, like storing data in the cloud. Detta knew exactly how to communicate things so as to minimize conflict and maximize her utility. Had this happened a decade ago, Detta would have coordinated it all. With her gone, the Good siblings have a little learning to do.

Dad hears from Clement and Libby first. They each respond with their own version of *"Of course, I will!"*

Paul, who checks his email quarterly, and probably from the library, responds a few weeks later. He agrees to the test, but he's not the kind of guy who uses exclamation marks.

Clement and Libby send their kits to Stanford quickly, and a week later, Dr. Levine calls to let Dad know that neither of them is a match. Paul hasn't sent his sample yet, but we anticipated he would do this on his schedule, if at all. We stop talking about the idea of a transplant for a while, and Dad seems relieved. Since he's always looked after his siblings, asking one of them to undergo a stem cell harvest is complicated for him. Maybe if doctors used a word that didn't conjure images of alien probings, Dad wouldn't have been quite so tentative.

A month passes, and though Dad continues to respond well to his treatment, Dr. Levine reminds him that chemotherapy is not a cure. We should try to enjoy the time it has given us, but not lose sight of the ticking clock.

———————

Dr. Levine started delaying each of Dad's chemo treatments to let his good white blood cells recover. As soon as his white-blood-cell count reaches the low/normal range, Dad gets the poison again. That's just how chemo works: though his leukemia is still in remission, it's important to keep his marrow honest, to thwart any plans it has of printing out more counterfeits. This extra recovery time gives Dad and Mom an opportunity to visit us a for week in June, which is a beautiful month in New Jersey. Warm but not yet muggy, it's perfect weather for the lizards, and we spend most of their visit outside on our back patio enjoying the sun.

"How you feeling, Dad?" I ask, as Mom sips from a Sunday afternoon glass of Trader Joe's wine.

"I feel great!" he answers, quickly, and without further detail. I imagine he's tired of the question. It only serves as a reminder to him that he's still sick.

He does seem to be back to his old self. He made a solo run to Costco for steaks and is busy grilling them to perfection: four minutes on one side, five on the other. We are all enjoying this return to normalcy.

While waving smoke from his face, Dad's phone rings. He wipes his hands on a paper towel, reaches into his back pocket and looks at it, appearing a bit confused. "Jesus, it's my goddamn dentist again."

"Again? You mean he's called you many times?" I ask.

Mom laughs. "It *is* pretty strange."

"I'm due for a cleaning. He calls me three times a week."

"I've never been contacted by a dentist in my life," I say.

Lindsay appears from inside the house. From what I can tell she's been busy negotiating a disagreement between Silas and Arlo over the ownership of a mini-trampoline in our basement. When they run off to compete over the coveted yellow swing instead, she collapses onto a chair next to Mom.

I tell her that Dad's dentist is stalking him.

"That's random. How so?"

"Calling him all the time."

"You mean like socially?" she asks. We all laugh.

I turn to Dad. "Okay, tell the truth. Is it really your dentist?"

Dad shows me his phone. The most recent call is from a contact named "Dentist."

"That doesn't prove anything. You created a contact name for that number. It could be a brothel. Let me listen to the message."

Dad plays it for me: "Hi, Michael, it's Dr. Freid's office reminding you that you're due for a cleaning. It's very important that you call us back immediately."

"Wow, it sounds urgent!" I say. "I haven't had my teeth cleaned in a decade."

"Me, neither," Lindsay adds, and then, with a frustrated hand wave, indicates that it's my turn to referee the yellow swing battle.

When I return, Dad's phone rings again.

"If that's your dentist, you need to get a restraining order," I say, but Dad had already answered and he waves me off. "Yes, hello, Dr. Levine." He sticks his index finger into his other ear, bending at the waist. Lindsay, Mom, and I tune in like safecrackers as Dad paces the patio.

". . . Okay. Yes, I suppose that is great news," Dad says. We endure a long, tortuous pause.

"Well, I'm in New Jersey visiting my son right now. Would it be okay if I call him when I return? . . . Seven days. Great. Thank you, Dr. Levine."

Then a final pause: "Yes, you too."

Expressionless, Dad puts his phone back in his pocket.

"WELL?" I say.

"Paul is a perfect bone marrow match."

"YES!" Mom shouts.

"So this means you can get a transplant?" Lindsay asks. She tries to stay up on everything, but "mommy brain" still handicaps her retention of facts. I'm glad she asked, though, because Dad's answer surprises me.

"Yes, it does. Of course, Paul has to agree to be the donor. And he has to go through a series of tests to see if he's healthy and fit enough for it."

"You don't seem excited," I say.

"We'll have to see how it all works out," he said, turning his attention back to the grill. "It might be too soon to get excited. I mean, this is an opportunity, but it's also a big risk. I'll have to think about it."

I'm sure Dad wants to be thrilled, but his wish to be eligible for a cure comes with the emotional complication of involving his youngest brother in the process. We don't discuss the issue much for the rest of the next week, but it's clear from Dad's demeanor that the decision weighs on him. To alleviate stress, he puts things off, claiming he can't do one thing until he completes something else first. But for this, waiting is too much of a gamble.

I'm also conflicted. As real as the inevitability of him dying in nine months was, so now is the possibility that he might survive. I had mentally prepared for the worst, and as it seemed that the worst might not play out as planned, I find myself confused and, almost disappointed, somehow let down, that my father might not die as scheduled. *How dare he get me all revved up for something terrible and then not deliver?*

Of course, I want him to be here forever. But his illness also brought good things into our relationship. I fear that I won't have to carry him out of a movie theater again (though he might let me as some kind of gag). I am melancholy that we've already stopped holding hands from time to time, and angry at the way Dad's condition weaved itself into our emotional lives in the same way it did his physical body. Blood tests, hemoglobin, lymphocyte, and neutrophil percentages are our conversational topics now. It's who we are.

It's as if we had been on an airplane together and, certain that it was falling out of the sky, we expressed new intimacies and related in deeper, more meaningful ways. But as the captain regained control, we reverted to old patterns—unharmed, unchanged, and no wiser.

In the beginning of this ordeal, all I felt was panic, but Dad's illness also gave me focus, a defined purpose, and a needed disruption in routine. In those first few months, I may have been tense, frightened, shocked, but I was also present. A sane mind can't live in crisis mode forever, though, and the ebbing of all that adrenaline has left me feeling too much like myself again.

So, I did all I could to replace those depleted brain chemicals by focusing on the situation with Paul.

After Dad and Mom returned to California, I check in with Dad via text.

Jason
Did you talk to Paul yet?

Dad
I emailed him and told him he was a match, yes.

Jason
What did he say?

Dad
He sent a one-line response: "I knew I was because I am."

Jason
Jesus. That's so Paul. He's like Mark Twain.

Dad
Or Yogi Berra.

Jason
So what's next?

Dad
I have to decide if I want to do this or not.

Jason
Right. Well?

<u>Dad</u>

Honestly, I don't know yet. If I can get five more good years by staying on this drug, why shouldn't I just do that?

<u>Jason</u>

Because no one knows if you can get five more years. It could be five more weeks. Right now this is all hypothetical until we know if Paul is up for it.

<u>Dad</u>

He is. I got an email from him. I'll forward it to you.

An hour later, Dad sent me this:

Jason,

For some reason, the email from Paul has disappeared. He said that he would do anything to improve the quality/quantity of my life and is definitely on board. He expressed a deep mistrust of "Western medicine."

This disease was mine alone and that was a source of great comfort for me. Now Paul is an integral part of it and I really don't like that. The more I learn about his role, the more I understand the depth of his commitment. I'll know more Friday.

Dad

Sent from my iPad

I can't let Dad go any further down this path, so I call him.

"If Paul asked you to do this for him, you would agree, right?" I ask.

"Without question," he responds.

"And if you told him you would, but then he chose not to get the procedure because he didn't want to make you an integral part of his illness, how would you feel?"

"I would insist," he answers. "It's what brothers do for each other."

"Then how is this any different?"

"Well . . ."

"Well, what?"

"I'm not him and he's not me."

"You mean, you don't think he feels protective of you the same way you feel protective of him?"

"I don't know what I mean, but I imagine that's probably part of it, yes."

"He's pure and healthy now, and you don't want any part of possibly ruining that?"

"Hadn't thought of it like that, but *now* I do," he says, laughing.

"Sorry."

"No, don't be. You just said it more simply than I could have. Why should an old dying man who hasn't taken very good care of himself even get this chance?"

"This isn't your fault," I say. "Would you do it if you were fifty?"

"Hell yes."

"So it's an age thing, too. Some people live to be ninety."

"I'm not going to live to be ninety, Jason."

"Clearly. I'm just saying that despite feeling like you haven't taken good care of yourself, you're still in way better shape than the vast majority of sixty-nine-year-old men in this country. Have you been to the mall lately? Comparatively, you're in your mid-fifties."

Facts, common sense, science; they aren't getting through to him. He will have to go through with the transplant despite feeling squirrely. The role of a donor is minimal and relatively painless. I think Dad exaggerates it because he needs an excuse to put off making a decision. There is no needle thrust into anyone's spine, no sucking out of viscous, yellow fluid. In fact, there's no actual marrow involved at all. The "harvesting" will be no more invasive than donating blood. Paul would be given a drug to encourage his bone marrow to make more stem cells, and those extra, "peripheral" stem cells will be collected from his blood. As I understand it (albeit, in pidgin science) they will hook Paul up to Dad like jumper cables to an old car, turn the ignition, and hope for the best.

Dad is standing on the ledge of a building. Behind him are the villains with guns, and below him, uncertainty. The transplant will throw his body into entropy, and given how good he feels, it's hard to agree to a procedure that will certainly make him awful. That is the conundrum: being in remission is the primary requirement for getting a transplant—a life-threatening procedure that, if successful, requires a six-month recovery period during which Dad must take the precautions of a first responder to an Ebola outbreak.

He will be forbidden from going outside, but if he does, he will have to wear a HEPA mask. Not the 3M cotton masks worn by overly cautious Chinese women on the New York subway. No, his will be like a hazmat helmet, the kind that makes people look like human anteaters on a government contract to clean up asbestos.

In the house, he can't be left alone. Mom can't go to the grocery store or to Curves for her sweatless workout. Someone will have to be with him at all times, probably me, Lindsay, or one of his siblings.

Perhaps the downstairs neighbor who smokes fish in an open oven at all times of the night could help, or maybe a random stranger off the street we pay ten dollars an hour to sit there and make sure Dad doesn't contract a spontaneous infection or fall and bleed to death while watching *CSI: Miami.*

He will have to refrain from entering a room for five minutes after it has been vacuumed because of dust.

Oh my God. THE DUST.

He can't touch meat, fresh fruit, or vegetables because of bacteria. *Holy shit, the bacteria.* He will be a man to whom the world has suddenly become poisonous.

There are other equally restricting guidelines, all of which I'm sure we will be able to bend eventually, but going in we have to prepare to follow them strictly. At a certain point, it's hard not to think, "Why the hell *would* he do this?" He's already almost seventy years old. How many good years does he have left? Is this any different from giving Mickey Mantle a new liver?

Dad has been deemed healthy enough for the procedure, but the chance that this will cure him is only 50 percent. No wonder he's tempted to just stay on his current chemo and hope for a miracle. Even if the transplant is successful—that is, if Dad's and Paul's immune systems don't have a full-out bar brawl over who was in charge—where will that put him? He might be cancer free, but at what cost? At what toll to his body and mind? At what toll to us as a family?

The alternative is equally ridiculous: staying on a relatively new drug, keeping his fingers crossed that it continues to work and does so longer than it was supposed to. But how long is long enough? What's an adequate number of years to wring out of life? Seventy-two? Seventy-five? Some people get half that.

We're in the casino again, facing people we don't know and games we don't quite understand. He has chips in his hand, but there is no safe bet. A 50 percent chance of being cured is also a 50 percent chance of not being cured, which will probably result in death from infection or via the charmingly named "graft-versus-host disease."

I've read about this. The writer Susan Sontag, who suffered from the same condition, demanded a transplant despite having only a partially matched donor. Her son published an essay in the *New York Times* about sitting by helplessly as his mother's body ate itself from the inside out. She died covered in sores and pustules, as if stricken by a medieval plague.

Thankfully, with Paul being a perfect match, we are in a slightly better situation. An acute rejection of the new stem cells is still possible but less likely. There is some counterintuitive science involved (I've learned that if science were intuitive, there wouldn't be scientists). Apparently, a little rejection is good. As Dad's immune system has a mild panic attack over the introduction of a new operating system, his body will kill off any remaining cancerous blood cells, like a startled blind man with a pistol shooting anything that makes a sound. It will be important that Dad's new immune system not get its hands on a bomb. Doctors manage this balance with drugs, something to calm his white blood cells, Xanax for the immune system, or so I imagine it.

Dad has been thinking a lot about this, too. He and Mom met with the transplant coordinator at Stanford. The team is ready for him; all they need is for Paul to come to Palo Alto and undergo a few tests to determine his suitability. But Dad told them that he had to think about it some more. Sometimes easy decisions are the most difficult to make.

Lizards

Under the spell of the evil spirit that convinces people to make big changes at odd times (one that seems to have possessed Dad when he was my age), Lindsay and I decided, during all this, to leave our little New Jersey village. It was a town for people who worked in Manhattan, not for a comedian-turned-writer and a modern-dancer-turned-full-time mom. Lindsay and I had discussed this move for months, and over the summer of 2013, we hired some brawny dudes to pack our East Coast life in bubble wrap, and move it to Minneapolis.

I would have pushed harder for Oakland, to be closer to Mom and Dad, but it was too expensive, and after dozens of visits I still didn't understand what people did in the Bay Area. It seemed like they spent most of their time parking, recycling, and determining the source of odd street smells.

Lindsay's sister, brother-in-law, their two kids, and Lindsay's mom all still live in Minneapolis. Lindsay went to high school in nearby Long Lake and has friends in the area. It's affordable and has good schools. Plus, it's a four-hour flight to Oakland, instead of the dreaded six from Newark. I saw Dad's illness as a temporary situation for all of us, anyway. I figured if he died, we'd move Mom to Minneapolis, at least season-ally. She wouldn't want to. She'd argue that she likes being alone. But I promised Dad that's what I would do. It's also possible that choosing Minneapolis over Oakland was a way for me to maintain some distance, to avoid becoming further consumed by Dad's illness. *My parents are in charge of their lives. I am in charge of mine.* They try to be supportive. "Sounds great to us! You'll have family around all the time," Mom says. "Of course, you'd have that here, too, but we understand."

"Do you have snowshoes yet?" Dad asks.

Mom updates her Facebook status to "Loving the sunlight and year-round 70 degree weather here!" I can't take it anymore, so I text her:

Jason

I saw your Facebook post about how beautiful everything is there. Are you trying to make me feel guilty?

Mom

Oh, God no! I was just really enjoying the weather! How's Minneapolis? Getting ready for winter?

Mom is unstoppable. When she emails me a real estate listing for a house near theirs, I respond, "Why did you send me this? We're not moving to Oakland."

"Oh, I know that! I just thought it was a pretty house."

"This one looks nice, too," I write back, attaching an advertisement for a villa in Spain.

She ignores it. "We'll have to come out for a visit before it gets too cold."

"It's July," I tell her. "You have plenty of time."

I can tell that Mom and Dad are unhappy about all this, but they would never say so out loud. They rarely expressed any forthright concerns or negativity about my decisions. In movies, there are often strange scenes where fathers and sons have tender, contemplative moments. These usually take place on a boat dock, in a wheat field, or on a baseball diamond—someplace manly and trite. The father gives his son a piece of sage advice that the son finds difficult to understand. Years later, when the boy has become a man, he faces a predicament, and summons that wisdom and perseveres. We're supposed to be touched, but I suspect we're all rolling our eyes because nobody's father ever does that.

I don't believe Mom and Dad are intentionally passive-aggressive. It's simply a side effect of holding in one's opinions. They released me into the wild when they moved to Italy in 1990. They tagged me and watched my movements, but never intervened. Perhaps, for them, my life has been one long, ongoing anthropological experiment.

Twenty years ago when I was distraught over the end of a five-year romantic relationship, Mom said, "Well, if it makes you feel better, Dad and I never liked her."

"I thought you loved Amy," I said. "She was so funny."

"Really? You thought she was funny?" Dad said. "She was mentally ill."

"What?"

"We were terrified you were going to marry her," Mom added.

"You should have told me that!"

"Would it have changed your mind about her?" Dad asked.

"No."

"Well, then, there you have it."

Maybe in addition to the setting, it's watching a son actually listen to his father that makes those movie scenes seem so absurd. Instead of telling me what to do, Dad learned it was more fruitful to plant seeds that made good choices easier to make.

In September, after settling into a new, cheaper, and Midwestern-sized home, the lizards come to see us. Thankfully, they make it before the temperature falls below fifty degrees, the point at which their trident-shaped tongues turn to icicles. Dad has been practicing his Minnesota accent, and uses it to quote Garrison Keillor ad nauseum. "So, are the men strong, the women good-looking, and all the children above average here?" He sounds more like Rick Moranis in *Strange Brew* than a Minnesotan.

Despite it being wonderfully crisp (warm enough for a light jacket in the evening and hot enough for short sleeves during the day), Mom and Dad pay the weather no compliments. Mom wraps herself in a shawl at 2 PM in silent protest. The leaves are orange and red, the maples still green. Our block is packed with kids named Beckett, Whitaker, Bennett, and so on. A few are already in their Halloween costumes, riding Razor scooters, and shooting each other with water pistols (and water semi-automatics). It's like the 1950s, but in color, and no one is named Gary or Patty.

Halfway through their two-week visit, I slink up from my office lair in the basement to make coffee. I hear Mom and Dad arguing in their room. It's technically the "master suite," but Lindsay and I have yet to use it because we sleep upstairs with the boys like a litter of kittens.

Mom and Dad sound tense, and I strain to hear specifics, but can only make out tone. As I put milk in my coffee, I hear Mom yell, "Get out of here! Just get out of here!"

I leave the milk on the counter and dash back to the stairs, but Dad walks in before I can escape. "Your mother's having one of her fits."

"Yeah? About what?" I answer in a fake, carefree voice.

"Oh, who the hell knows? She says she wants to be alone, so I left her alone. You should go talk to her if you're feeling brave."

I find Mom pacing the bedroom, and walk past her to sit in the chair underneath the window. I'm a sit-first-and-ask-questions-later kind of man.

"Hi," she says. "Sorry you had to hear all that." Her face is red, hands trembling a bit.

"I didn't hear much. What's going on?"

"Every time we come here I say we should stay no more than two weeks. Then your father makes the reservations himself and it's always for longer. I know you guys don't want us here for that long. I'm sure Lindsay doesn't want us here for longer than two weeks, but your father just thinks we can stay as long as we want, and I just don't like it. There's nothing for me to do here. I can't go to Curves, and I can't even go for a walk because I don't know the neighborhood very well..."

Dad was right, she is having a fit.

"Mom, you guys can stay as long as you want, but I totally under-stand if *you* don't want to stay this long."

"You do?" She seems pleasantly surprised.

"I live here and don't want to stay for two weeks sometimes. It's chaos. Come back here to your room and read whenever you want. Everyone needs a break now and then."

"See, Dad doesn't get that. He doesn't understand that I could want to be alone. He made me promise not to read while I'm here because it's antisocial. But he watches so much TV! Isn't that worse?"

"Well, he grew up in chaos. You and I didn't."

"You're right. He likes it when everyone is talking over the TV. That's exactly what his house was always like."

"And nothing makes us more uncomfortable."

"Yes!"

These meltdowns happen once or twice a year. Mom holds a lot in. When I try to talk with her about Dad's condition, ask her how she's feeling, she always turns it back on me by asking how *I* am feeling. Then she agrees with whatever I say. Dad has always argued that he and I are complicated and weak, and Mom is simple and strong. He means it as a compliment to all of us (I've argued, unsuccessfully, that he and I are indeed weak, but also simple). Maybe Mom doesn't need to talk about things so much. I remember how stoic and focused she was when her father died. It wasn't until she saw him in the funeral home—still and waxen—that she broke down. Her reaction was intense but short, like she'd decided to somehow let her emotions build up, release them in one ninety-second burst, and then never speak of it again.

I map out a couple of walking routes for her to our local downtown area, where there's an Anthropologie, a Sur La Table, and a few boutiques. "I'll deal with Dad," I tell her. For the rest of the visit, *she* chooses when to play with Silas and Arlo. That is, she appears only when the kids aren't being a pain in the ass. That is the advantage to being a grandparent: you can disappear when the screaming starts.

After his argument with Mom, Dad checks out, and spends the subsequent seven days watching CNN, going to Costco, and using every pot in the house to cook elaborate meals. No one trashes a kitchen like an amateur chef who knows he won't have to clean up.

I always assumed that responsible "grown-ups" had good reasons for their behavior. By the time I turned thirty, I realized that adults are seldom driven by rational choice, but rather by mysterious forces that only psychologists and psilocybin mushrooms can sort out.

Instead of growing up, we simply become more aware of how ridiculous we are and learn to hide it. Maturing is nothing more than accepting how full of shit you are. A side effect of this is the realization that everyone else is full of shit, too, including your parents. It's almost frightening that these flawed, ridiculous human beings were once in charge of feeding me and guiding me in the ways of the world.

I spent most of my life emulating Dad, but now, as I've limped from his shadow, I realize that I am not as much like him as I thought. I'm simply a combination of two very different people with a handful of miscellaneous, semi-functioning parts mixed in, just like everyone else.

As I transition from the immediate gratification (and sometimes horror) of stand-up comedy, to the delayed gratification (and relentless horror) of writing, I see how similar I am to Mom. In a subconscious, pre-emptive strike in the emotional battle of a future without Dad, my connection with her has grown over the past year. There's no one else in the world with whom I feel more comfortable being silent. We've been emailing each other articles about the power of introverts, as well as various tests to determine one's level of social comfort. She dislikes people more than I do, but it's a close contest.

Socializing feeds Dad.

It depletes Mom and me. We're both only children and value our alone time.

Dad hates being alone.

Mom and I hate small talk.

Dad loves it.

Mom understands when to let me be, but Dad has a knack for wanting to bond or chat at times when I'm burrowed deepest in my hole.

Mom always seems content. "She lives life so perfectly," Dad has said. Aside from her beauty, Mom rarely makes a lasting first impression. She's a wallflower, forced from the comforts of solitude by a lifelong partner who wants to party all the time. One must read a few chapters of Mom before getting sucked in, but Dad is an open book with a worn-out binding and Post-it notes smattered throughout: *Here I am, everyone. Love me or hate me. Hurry up, I'm waiting!*

Many of Dad's biggest laughs at parties come from repeating something Mom just muttered under her breath. On the rare occasion that she protests Dad's blatant hacking of her best lines, he argues, "Well, Jody, you should have said it louder."

This is one of the reasons they've stayed together so long. Two socially boisterous people would fight with each other for attention. Mom lets Dad have all of it. When two introverts partner for life, they often end up accumulating too many cats and become buried under trade periodicals.

An hour or so after my talk with Mom, I'm in my office, trying to write, but become distracted by my frustrations with Dad. It's been over three months since we found out Paul was a match. Had Dad done the transplant immediately, he could be cured by now.

Dad knocks on the door. I know it's him, because everyone else in my family barges in like they're reporting a fire.

"So what was going on with your mom?" he asks, perhaps feeling a little repentant.

"She just wants to be alone."

"But this is her family. How could she not want to be with her *family?*"

"That's kind of what being alone means." I tell him. "If other people are around, regardless of their relation to you, then you're not alone."

"Well, as long as you understand it."

"If you want to be with your family so badly, maybe you should call Stanford and tell them you're ready to do the transplant." My nervous system is on high alert now. I probably shouldn't have said that.

Dad stares at me for a few seconds and then slaps my desk. "Yup, that's what I'm going to do." Is this what he's been waiting for? For me to just come out and tell him what to do. Why did I wait so long?

At the end of Mom and Dad's visit, we speak briefly about Thanksgiving. They invite us to come out to San Leandro, but given that it is our first holiday in our new city, and we are surrounded—flanked, really—by Lindsay's family, we decide to stay. Of course, there is *no chance* of Mom and Dad risking their lives to come to Minneapolis for what is sure to be an arctic November.

Cockroach

The night before Thanksgiving, Silas nestles up, waiting for me to read him a bedtime story.

"What are you doing on your phone?" he asks.

"Texting with BooBoo," I answer.

"Why?"

"He's not feeling well."

"Oh, he's sick again? And that's why you're going there?"

"Well, yes. I mean, he's been sick this whole time. He was feeling better for a while, but now he's even sicker." It's not easy to explain the concept of remission and relapse to a child.

"Is he going to die?" Silas asks.

"Not really soon, but maybe."

His eyes well up. "Well, there will still be Mimi," he says, turning his head away.

"Oh, honey. It's okay to cry."

Silas quickly wipes his eyes. "*I wasn't crying.*" He scowls at me, an adorable kid version of Jack Nicholson in *The Shining*.

"Oh, it looked like you were about to," I say. "It's okay if you do."

"Well, I wasn't. Whatever." He pauses, collects himself, and asks, "Would you cry if BooBoo died?"

"Of course."

"Like for two whole days?"

"Well, not two days straight, but I'd cry a lot for a long time. But we don't need to talk about this right now unless you want to." It isn't the right time to explain the grieving process to a six-year-old. In my mind, I've already abdicated that responsibility to Lindsay. I have to remember to tell her that.

"Okay," he says, snapping back into a good mood. When is it exactly that we lose such emotional resilience?

"We still have to read the last chapter of that *Secrets of Droon* book," I say.

"Oh yeah! *And* I have to return it to the library tomorrow so we have to finish it tonight."

"Okay, then. Chapter ten, 'A Spell from the Past.'"

A year after being diagnosed, five months after going into remission, and two months after slapping my desk in determination, Dad finally pulled the trigger. Four days before, he had told Stanford he was ready to move forward with the bone marrow transplant. Forty-eight hours after that, his weekly blood test hinted that the drugs had stopped working. A bone marrow biopsy confirmed that the fruits of Dad's faulty marrow were more bitter than before. His cancer had mutated and progressed to AML (acute myeloid leukemia). The transplant that had been penciled in for December 29 was canceled. The upside? We learned that time is not something to fuck with.

AML was Dad's original diagnosis, the same that spurred our emergency trip to California the previous year. Dr. Levine recanted a few days later in favor of a softer diagnosis. There was no ambiguity now. Dad's only option (aside from a "natural death") was to get the very chemotherapy that Dr. Levine had avoided for fear it would kill him.

On Thanksgiving Day, I flew out alone to California. Dad expressed concern over the boys seeing him in the hospital, as well as exposing them to all the plagues wafting about the halls. Lindsay thought seeing BooBoo might be good for them. She'd recently read that bearing witness to life's cycle helps kids understand the impermanence of all things, that sickness and death are normal, inevitable, and not to be feared. I thought that instead of teaching the boys this lesson via the terminal illness of their grandfather, perhaps we should ease them into it more slowly by buying them a goldfish. It's best to teach kids reality in small increments.

Dad took a calculated risk by putting off the transplant. It is a difficult thing to give up, feeling good, even when we know we harbor a dormant disease that might wake up at any moment. Fear and denial fueled his hesitancy, but it also might have been his way of maintaining some control over a situation he knew would one day render him helpless.

The chemotherapy treatment Dad is about to get will drop his white-blood-cell count to zero. Though "targeted," the drug makes a lot of mistakes. In the process of killing rapidly dividing cancer cells, the rest of the blood cells, even the good ones, will be destroyed as collateral damage. Chemotherapy is a focused idiot.

In the face of this sudden turn, Dad seems calm, something he's incapable of faking. The tempered rage he expressed at Radio Shack is gone. Maybe this is an example of the *real stress* he has always sought— the kind that allows him to write off all the trifling stuff.

Dad does have something going for him that he didn't last November. Should he achieve another remission, a donor is waiting for him. Paul will join us for that part of the journey, like SP did when we went to Italy. Paul isn't as enthusiastic as SP was to accompany us, but for some reason, the universe thinks that Mom, Dad, and I need company when making big changes. Maybe it has a sense of humor or thinks the three of us are too tightly woven and in need of alternate perspectives. My guess is that it's just payback for all of our wisecracks about yoga and oolong tea. I imagine Lindsay would agree. It's karma.

The situation is different for me, too. I feel no panic this time. After absorbing the right hook of Dad's mortality, this jab leaves me merely stunned. My focus of late has been on my immediate family and our future—a future with or without Dad. I didn't consciously choose this shift. I don't have that kind of control over my thoughts. Instead, the gray matter in my brain has been slowly turning to mortar, and access to my emotions seems blocked by a brick wall: still there, but in the background, lingering in the crevices of my mind like bad credit. I'm told that turning off like this is a form of coping.

The patient coordinator has vouchers for Mom and me. "You can take these down to the cafeteria for your Thanksgiving dinner," he says, handing us pieces of paper with pictures of turkeys wearing pilgrim hats.

His name is Keith, big guy, high voice, probably an ex-football player. I call him "Big Keith," but not to his face.

At home in the tundra, Lindsay and the boys are together with their cousins, aunt, uncle, grandmother, and everyone else I'm related to by marriage. I'm glad I can be with Mom and Dad, and the weather is gorgeous—about sixty degrees warmer—but I wish we could all be together in Minneapolis instead. Lindsay tells me my brother-in-law said a prayer for us at the table. He comes from a good Christian family, the kind that doesn't judge us pagans too harshly. When I tell Dad, he smiles and says, "Well, it can't hurt."

On our way down to the mess hall, Mom and I pass packs of cackling nurses and residents, each of them holding a brown Styrofoam box of holiday slop. I feel like we're extras in an episode of some hospital show, mere foils for the comedic repartee of the witty, wacky staff.

Mom and I didn't know the hospital would be providing meals, so the night before went to Whole Foods to get turkey, mashed potatoes, and all the other fixin's. We planned on heating them up using the microwave at the nurses' station outside Dad's room. He requested that we bring oyster stuffing, saying, "Like my mom used to make." It's a putrid, squishy culinary miasma that might have been invented by an alcoholic railroad tycoon wearing a monocle and top hat. Mom and I rolled our eyes.

At Whole Foods, we realized we hadn't eaten since breakfast and opted to hit the hot food bar before taking a number at the "Thanksgiving Deli." It was late, around 8 PM, and the seating area looked like a bus station: napkins strewn on the floor, the faint smell of rotten milk, students nearby hunched over cheap laptops. We found a dry table, sat down, and ate in silence. Chicken wings and macaroni and cheese for me; a broccoli-and-red-onion medley for Mom. Neither of us had the energy to discuss it, but we were practicing for life without Dad. It was pleasant—soothing, even—but not as fun.

In Dad's pale blue cell, the three of us struggle to make enough room for our meals on his rolling table/desk. On the side of it, there's a retractable mirror operated by a button that reads "release vanity." Since Dad's ass is visible almost constantly, releasing vanity seems like a good idea. It doesn't matter how tightly one ties the bottom strings of a hospital gown, they're designed for checking out a patient's backside as they shuffle by.

We move the iPad, laptop, and germ mask over to the small counter by the sink next to the closet. Dad sits on the side of his bed, an IV in his chest with a catheter threaded down next to his heart. The body's built-in pump is the most effective way to deliver the nasty stuff through the bloodstream. Dad hasn't figured out how to navigate all his cords, wires, and tubes yet.

"Jesus, do you think they could have me hooked up to more shit here?" he says.

"The bitter marionette. That would be a good character," I joke. I don't think Dad hears me, though. He's staring mutely at his meal: tuna salad on a croissant with a few pieces of melon and a cookie. "Why the hell do I get tuna?" he asks. Mom responds by donating her box. She would only have eaten the salad anyway.

"So, do you think this new chemo will make your hair fall out?" I ask, shoving a hillock of mashed potatoes into my mouth.

Dad runs his fingers through his hair. "This is the diesel stuff, Jace. I imagine it probably will."

"I read it's uncommon with cytarabine," I say.

"The other drug with a ridiculous name is the one that will make me lose it."

"Right." For the first time I feel like Dad knows more about his treatment than I do. "You should just shave your head now and start referring to yourself as Heisenberg."

"Good idea," he said. "I'll need a hat, though."

"Have you puked yet?" I ask.

"Jason, we're eating."

"Right, sorry. It's not bad, is it?"

"Oh, it's bad. I barely have the energy to stand up."

"No, I mean the food."

"Oh, the food. Yes, it's actually pretty good."

"The salad and melon are delicious!" Mom adds. Dad and I wink at each other in disbelief that anyone could like melon more than gravy.

A tall nurse with short, spiky blonde hair enters the room. She compliments Dad on his pajama bottoms (he ditched the gown). "I like the frogs on those. Very cute!"

"Thanks. I guess you could say I'm half asleep in frog pajamas." Dad waits to see if she gets the Tom Robbins reference.

She doesn't.

"Do you know the author Tom Robbins?" he asks.

"No, I don't think I do," she responds, unaccustomed to having this kind of conversation with patients.

"He wrote *Even Cowgirls Get the Blues*. It became a movie. Sissy Hankshaw? Uma Thurman played her. Big thumbs? Well, he also wrote a book called *Half Asleep in Frog Pajamas*."

"Oh, I'll have to read that, then, won't I?" She thinks Dad is weird, but she'll learn to like him soon enough. All the nurses will. Dad's main goal is to be popular in the hospital. It's the only part of this he can control.

Dad's doctors remain cryptic about his prognosis. They don't want to overpromise and underdeliver. "Yes, this is completely normal. Everything is fine and going according to plan," they say repeatedly. Often, I wonder if they are paying as close attention as we are.

"Why don't you get more details from them?" I ask Dad.

"Because they're busy and have other patients to see. I guess I like being taken care of, but I don't like being a problem."

"Jesus. You realize I understand everything now, right?" I ask.

"How so?"

"Your frustration and anxiety. It's all because you don't like being a problem."

"You think?"

"You don't?"

"I'm not doing a lot of thinking at all these days."

"Of course," I respond, a little embarrassed.

After we finish eating, I offer to replace the dog poster hanging on the wall. Dad hates dogs. "Why do people allow animals to live in their homes?" he's said.

"I could get that Florence cityscape from your kitchen."

"No, that's okay," he says, always the perfect patient. "Maybe I'll end up liking dogs."

Because I don't want to be the kind of person who insists that a hospital room be decorated according to its tenant's tastes, I let it go.

I can't do anything physically, or intellectually, to help here. Emotional support is my role, and Mom and Dad can't stop thanking me. "Jeez, we just don't know what we would do if you weren't here with us for all this." I find it hard to accept that my mere presence is enough. At home with my family, I'd become accustomed to a more hands-on, creative kind of caretaking. The prior month I had to hold Arlo down while a pediatric dentist did a "drill and fill" on one of his molars. I started singing the ABCs to calm him. It was a desperate move, but it seemed to work. When Dr. Charlie (as he referred to himself) joined in, and then so too the hygienist, I became self-conscious and stopped.

Mom and I are quiet driving back from the hospital. There's no music, no GPS, no singing, no sense of relief. We spent hours sitting by Dad's side, fidgeting in the uncomfortable visitors' chairs. I know he will be fine for the evening by himself. Doug, a former student of Dad's who fell backward into piles of money, brought him a new iPad Air and a Verizon LTE hotspot. The Internet connection is so slow at the hospital that I told Dad he could use the hotspot password like cigarettes in prison: "You know, to get things you need from other patients."

"Like what?" he asked.

"I don't know. An extra dinner roll?"

"With a shiv in it?"

"Sure, why not?"

When Mom and I arrive back at the penthouse, Dad's absence is heavy. It feels strange in here. Empty. Until this moment, I hadn't realized how much space Dad takes up—his presence, consciousness, and girth of personality fills this place. We don't mention it, but the idea that he might never return weighs on us. Mom sits in her chair, and I lie down on the sofa, both of us staring at our iPads.

"Have you read *Lolita*?" I ask.

"The one about the little girl and the adult man?"

"Yeah. Can I read you the first two paragraphs?"

"Sure." Mom loves being read to.

Lo-lee-ta: the tip of the tongue taking a trip of three steps down the palate to tap, at three, on the teeth. Lo. Lee. Ta. . . .

"Incredible, right?"

"Yuppers," she says, distracted. If Dad were here, I imagine him having a bigger reaction. "Jesus Christ. Who the hell writes like that?!" he'd say, shaking his head in disbelief that anything could be so good. Maybe what we are missing is enthusiasm.

I try a little harder to engage Mom. "Did I send you that article about Dorothy Parker stealing Nabokov's story and publishing a piece in the *New Yorker*?"

"Oh yes, you did. I'd forgotten. I think she was on her way down at that point. I just can't believe she kept the same title."

"I know. I think it was a deniability thing. Like, 'Hey, if I were going to steal something, don't you think I'd be smart enough to at least change the title and the name of the main character?'"

"Oh, you're probably right." Mom still seems disinterested. I picked the wrong time to pretend like everything is normal.

"Okay, I'm heading off to bed. I'm pooped," she says.

"Yeah, long day. See you in the morning. I love you."

"I love you, too." She smiles. "We'll get through this."

"I know."

I stay on the sofa and continue to read *Lolita*, imagining how Dad might react to some of the passages. Soon after Mom turns out her light, I receive a text message from Dad.

Dad

The nurse just gave me morphine. This is going to be good, isn't it?

Jason

Why do you need morphine?

Dad

She asked if I was in any pain, and I said, "Does existential pain count?"

Jason

Hilarious. And she gave it to you?

Dad

Well, I had a bit of a back spasm too.

Jason

So jealous. Was it IV?

Dad

Yeah, buddy. Already feeling it.

I search YouTube for the Louis CK bit about opiate suppositories. It's one of my favorites. Nearly a year has passed since I've performed stand-up, and I am finally able to enjoy comedy again as a fan. In the clip, Louis tells Conan O'Brien how difficult it was for him to put the opium up his ass, but how amazing it felt when he finally found the courage.

I text the link to Dad, but don't hear anything back for a few minutes.

Jason

Did you get that link?

Dad

Yes. Lifting so hard I'm faking.

Jason

WHAT?

Dad

Sorry laughing using Siri for tests. Texts I mean. Fuck you Siri.

Jason

Oh, good. I thought you were so high that you couldn't type.

Dad

I can't. Why do you think I used it description with? Man, this is some good shit.

Dad is hammered, and I couldn't be more pleased about it. He's certainty earned some sweet opiate relief. I'm also pleased to see that Siri now understands curse words better than she does verbs. Maybe the slurred speech helps somehow.

Thirty years ago, I remember Dad being in a similar state. His doctor had prescribed him Vicodin for a kidney stone. He was upstairs, and kept calling for me from his bed, like a Victorian aristocrat after a fainting spell. I was uninterested in stopping whatever inane thing eleven-year-olds do on weekend afternoons at home. He kept calling, his voice getting weaker and weaker. Finally, I approached the top of the stairs, peered into Mom and Dad's bedroom, and saw him lying there in his underwear, his face covered in Bag Balm, a boutique version of Vaseline—that thick, greasy, clear jelly crap no one should ever use.

"Dad?" I said.

"Hey Jace! My boy!" he slurred. "I just wanted you to see what your Dad looks like when he's reaaaaallly fucked up."

"Oh, okay," I said. "What's that stuff all over your face?"

"Bag Balm, Buddy! You wanna try some? Feels good to just smear it around."

"No, thanks."

"Suit yourself, sport," he said and closed his eyes.

I imagine him like that now, only this time, yelling into an iPad and laughing uncontrollably. I head off to bed, happy.

Roadside Distractions

The next morning, Mom and I sit at the breakfast bar in the apartment drinking coffee. "You heard from Dad yet this morning?" I ask.

"Oh yes! He's been texting me since seven, asking when we were coming today."

"Does he expect us to be there all day every day?"

"Oh, I don't know. He probably does. It's just so boring. You know he doesn't like being alone. Even when he's in his den, he talks to the TV like it's a person."

"You mean he yells at it?"

"Yes, there's that. But he also carries on a dialogue sometimes."

"A dialogue?"

"If he's watching a show on MSNBC, he'll talk as if he's one of the panelists."

"There's something very sad and hilarious about that. We should probably head over soon, right?"

"I'm ready when you are."

On our way out, I rear back and jack Bozo in his fat red nose. He falls, and then pops right up again. Just like depression. Just like cancer. What a dick.

When we arrive in Dad's room, Mom and I learn why he'd been rushing us. The night before, while floating in his pleasant morphine haze, Dad's brother, Clement, had copied him on an email thread. Dad had yet to tell his siblings that he'd relapsed and the transplant was off.

"You should read this," Dad says, turning his laptop around so we could see the screen. "I don't know if he sent this to me on purpose or not, but it's not good."

Paul, Dad's youngest brother and bone marrow match, wrote:

When it's said that Mick is scheduled for his transplant, I realize I'm just a pawn in Stanford's game. I also realize that Mick is the main character in this drama and is compelled by the sovereign instinct to choose life at any cost.

I think, "what about my life?"

Then I think, "my life" isn't on the line.

None of the above, however, addresses the real question, which is whether or not a bone marrow transplant should even be on the table.

Gayle, as you might imagine, is struggling with it. She's asked if Jason's blood's been tested, if cord blood was collected when his two children were born, if Mick would be willing to go ahead if any of them were involved. Perhaps these are also questions that need to be asked.

I'm confused, furious, and unhinged by my aunt's dismissiveness. "Is Gayle really suggesting that Dad would ask Paul to donate but not me or Silas or Arlo? Does she think Dad has some list of people who might be eligible donors that he color-coded based on how important each of them is to him, and Paul's at the bottom?"

Mom and Dad are giving me a long leash. They can tell I need to stretch my legs. "I don't understand," I continue. "This is what people *do* for each other. Aren't there anonymous donors out there, too? Those people are willing to do it for anyone, but Gayle doesn't want Paul to do it for his fucking brother? Don't they understand if it were plausible that the boys or I were matches that we would have been tested? And if, by random chance, we were matches, that I would insist on donating?"

"Of course you would." Mom is always on my side, even when I'm being a lunatic. "They are both just so backward about all this," she says. "It's crazy." Finding it cathartic, Mom and I take this opportunity to focus our anger on people rather than on a nebulous disease. It feels quite therapeutic.

"I bet there are more emails," I say, as if researching a crime.

Mom plays along. "You think?"

"Yeah, there have to be. No way did the conversation end there." I'm eager to dig into the mysterious, possibly scheming, minds of my aunt and uncle. So much so that I lose sight of what's important: Dad. This is another drama for me to focus on—a fire escape.

Dad calls Clement that afternoon, and he admits to sending the email accidentally. "I guess I'm so used to sending stuff to all of you that I did it out of habit," he says. "I was thinking you should have been in the loop about all this, anyway. I was praying either Libby or I would be a match. I knew it would be complicated with Paul."

Paul's deep mistrust of Western medicine percolated while he waited for Dad's decision. Agreeing to donate must have been easy for Paul when it seemed so far in the future, but as the dates came into focus, and Stanford called him to schedule preliminary tests, Paul balked.

A few minutes later, Clement forwards Dad another email. This one from Gayle. The three of us read it together.

Libby and Clement,

I am starting this with you because I know Mick and Jody have their hands full right now. I am not on board right now with Paul being a donor. The process has health risks for him and NO ONE is answering the questions we have been asking for months. He has never had a complete physical or any health tests and we do not prescribe to general western medicine practices. You all know this about us and yet no one is acknowledging it.

Paul has spent his life preventing illness by attention to wellness, good diet and exercise. To just assume he would subject himself to this and all the possible side effects and risks is uncaring. We also currently have no health insurance and are reluctant to get involved with a system we don't like and can't afford . . .

So unless somebody starts to acknowledge our concern, there could be great disappointment on many levels.

Gayle

I pace Dad's hospital room, stepping over cords, and weaving my way past various beeping things on wheels. I want to knock them over, just clear the room like fed-up people on TV. "If Paul and Gayle had so many concerns, why didn't they come to us for answers? I could have told them that Dad's insurance covers all of the donor's medical costs."

"Is that right, Michael?" Mom asks.

Dad looks away. "Yes, I believe it is."

"So they think you should go ahead and die?" I ask. "And what's this shit about you *assuming* he would do this? *You asked him and he already agreed!* Do they have any idea how hard it was for you to even ask them to get their blood tested? You're also uncaring? What the fuck is going on?"

Dad is quiet. I figure he's disappointed or has perhaps given up.

I take a few deep inhales from my e-cig, which calms me a bit. Dad finally provides his thoughts. "Look, the last thing I heard directly from Paul is that he'd do anything to increase the quality and quantity of my life. He and Gayle have every right to express their doubts to whomever they like in any way they like. Unless he tells me himself that he's not willing to donate, I'm going to assume he still is."

How is it possible, that among the three of us, Dad is the rational one? He thinks it's best not to become secretly involved in other people's business. Even when their business is you. Of course, he's right, but it's difficult to find satisfying things to talk about when the private lives of others are off the menu.

Though Dad and I are in a period of confluence, the biological hierarchy of wisdom remains intact. Beyond our understanding, friendship, and camaraderie, he's still my father. We love Paul and Gayle, and respect how they've chosen to live their lives, but we also know it hasn't always been a choice. Unable to afford health insurance, perhaps they had merely embraced (maybe a bit too tightly) the options within their budget. An outsider might consider all of us brainwashed—Paul and Gayle by the holistic culture, and us by the Western Medicine Industrial Complex. Then again, as astrophysicist Neil deGrasse Tyson says, "The great thing about science is that it's true whether or not you believe in it."

Because Mom and I are high school girls, we convince Dad to send out a feeler to Paul, like passing him a note in class. We don't know if he knows that we know how he feels or if he knows that we've seen these emails. We would be better off not knowing any of this is going on. I guess this is what happens when people over the age of sixty-five use computers.

Dad emails Paul a short update about his condition. "Had another round of chemo. The strong stuff this time. Tired and bald. Look like G. Gordon Liddy, but feeling better every day." Paul responds quickly (for him), saying he's happy that Dad is "on the mend" and that he will send him "a ball cap."

I imagine Paul is still hoping the transplant won't happen. Of course, he knows if it doesn't, Dad will die, and he obviously doesn't want that. I think he's stuck in a paradox similar to that of climate change. "What do we have to do to reverse it?" "Really? No, I'm sorry. I can't do that. I'll take my chances that something else will solve it."

I can't help but imagine Silas and Arlo in a similar situation: one of them terminally ill and in need of a transplant from the other. As much as they fight now over the ownership of swings, trampolines, and random pieces of plastic, I like to think each, when old enough, would agree to help the other without question.

In an effort to understand Paul's position, I consider how I might react if the situation were reversed—if I were on Paul's end of what I consider a bizarre, risky, and overzealous treatment. I'm just as afraid of alternative medicine as he is of its Western foil. The mere thought of an enema makes me nauseated and panicked. The few times I've taken echinacea, I'm fairly certain it made me sicker. If I get malaria, I'm taking all available pharmaceuticals even if local mythology suggests that the bark of a cinchona tree is equally effective and less toxic.

A cure for Dad's condition can only come from science, and I am completely committed to it. But I must consider how I might feel if one of my cousins moved to a distant island to join a bizarre cult and sent a letter telling me that he was sick and that my participation in concocting a lifesaving witch's brew was crucial.

Sad and strange, but how could I not read on?

Down the page, I read that the main ingredient in this potion is the middle toe of a relative, and of all seventeen cousins, only mine will suffice because none of the others has a purple aura.

It's awkward now, and though I'd likely write back, tentatively agreeing, I would do so only because I like my cousin and hope that more reasonable options might come along between now and the ceremony. Maybe he'll come to his senses, or his tribe will source a more local toe.

Then, some months later, after I've vanquished the thoughts of my toe being used in a stew, I receive a new letter: "Greetings! It was so nice of you to offer your toe. I need it in three weeks. You will have to come here, so our leader can cut it off with a boar's tooth. I hope that's not too much trouble."

Panicked that somehow my bluff of support has been called, I might email the other cousins to see what they think about this plan, whether they know anything about boars, and specifically if their teeth are an effective tool for toe removal. I would pay this request its due diligence. It's what we do for our families.

This absurd fantasy isn't even close to being a fair comparison, but it helps me not be angry anymore. I need that more than I need accuracy. To reinforce my commitment to a modern, Western cure for Dad, I have to marginalize the alternatives as best I can, cast them as silly witchcraft.

But there's another, more appropriate, aspect to this allegory. What if I felt deep in my bones that my cousin was being led astray by his tribe and this toe stew would hurt him rather than help him?

To Paul and Gayle, Western medicine is a corporate-driven enterprise that profits on people's fear of death, all while ignoring, perhaps even covering up, the easier, safer, lifestyle-based ways to stay healthy. They don't want Dad becoming a victim of it. Modern medicine can prolong life, but often at great cost and often at the expense of someone's quality of life. This is what Paul meant when he questioned whether the transplant should be on the table at all. To him, there is quality in a natural death.

"Sure, but he's not the one dying," Dad says. "Believe me, it changes your whole perspective. I look at these beautiful little boys and just can't imagine not doing everything I can to be around to watch them grow up."

"And you get no similar feeling when looking at a picture of me?" I asked.

Dad smirks. "Nope, not a thing."

In December, after I had been back in Minneapolis for a few weeks, Dad texts me about a message he received from his social worker, Susan.

Dad

Susan said she saw something on my chart about coordinating a call with Stanford. That has to be good news, right?

Jason

I don't see how it couldn't be. Why else would they be calling Stanford unless it was to tell them you were in remission and ready for the transplant?

Dad

That's exactly what I was thinking.

Yet again, we are jumping the gun and reading too much into too little information. When Stanford calls the next day, it's not what we expected. Nurse Herbach was thrilled to inform Dad that they'd found two anonymous donors: both perfect matches. After a little prying, they told him that Paul might have some complicating factors rendering him ineligible to donate. Dad didn't ask for details.

Lacking real information about why Paul was now considered an ineligible donor, we fill the void with more speculation. Mom and I are powerless against the adrenaline-releasing drama of What Might Be Going On. Had Paul made up some condition to get himself off the hook? (That's what I would have done in his position.) Or had he told them flat out he wouldn't do it? Had the transplant coordinators at Stanford decided their lives would be easier if they found someone who actually wanted to be part of the Western Medicine Industrial Complex? Perhaps the complicating factor was simply that Paul is too old. But no, if that were true, Stanford would never have bothered testing him in the first place.

For weeks, perhaps a month, we waste our energy on this. Then again, I wonder what else we would have talked about instead. Normally, Dad and I would ponder a question, and Mom would Google the answer before we had any fun with it. "What was that movie Gene Hackman won an Oscar for?"

Thirty seconds later Mom would chirp, "I think you mean *The French Connection*. But he didn't win. It says here on IMDB that . . ."

"Great! What the hell are we supposed to talk about now?" Dad would say.

I miss those conversations. Given how little time we have left together, I hate that we spent so much of it wondering what someone else is thinking. All the conjecture about doctor's opinions, what Paul and Gayle think, and what Paul might decide, is a roadside distraction— a set of cognitive stimuli that only slows us down and takes our eyes off the road. It's how we cope with our collective helplessness. We can't solve anything, but feeling like we *know stuff* gives us peace of mind.

By the middle of December, we hadn't heard from Paul in nearly a month. For much of that time, he was in New Zealand attending a buskers' festival. Why is there a buskers' festival, but more important, how do people afford to travel to New Zealand on a busker's wages?

Finally, Dad receives an email from Paul that answers all of our questions:

Mick,

I want to apologize for being so out of touch lately. It doesn't mean I haven't been thinking of you. It's quite the contrary actually. While I've been involved with my current travels and preparations for them, which have long been in the making, I have not forgotten that your life is consumed by your battle . . . and that you've entrusted yourself to the people at Stanford.

My communications with them began almost five months ago when I sent a letter to the hospital that I expect got lost in the shuffle. At any rate, I didn't get a reply. I later included the text of that letter in my first of several emails to Nurse Veronica Herbach. She had called me, as you said she would, to see if I had any questions. I told her I had a lot of questions and we agreed that email was an acceptable way to communicate.

Eventually, she arranged a phone call for me with Doctor Kutsami just before Christmas. Doctor Kutsami had read my previous communications with Nurse Herbach. I told her how my initial questions were about the procedure—how long would it take, how much of the drug would I get, what are the possible side effects and complications, what about my lack of health insurance—but since I had done some fairly extensive research of my own, with help from the Internet and several knowledgeable friends, my questions were about what other more viable and better options might be available to you.

I have felt from the very beginning that the age factor is significant. I know there are successful outcomes for patients even older than you are and that's encouraging. Nonetheless, we are both at added risk because of our age. As my conversation with Doctor Kutsami unfolded, we talked openly about the age issue. Here is some of what she said . . .

"Historically, the age limit for donors was 50, but we've since moved forward from that . . . Older siblings, however, show a higher risk of co-morbidities and just because you're a match it doesn't make you a donor. . . . It's not uncommon for a physician/advocate to decide, for a wide variety of reasons, that it's not appropriate for a matching sibling to be a donor. . . . Nurse Herbach has already started an unrelated donor search. If a good donor is found in the database, it will be nearly as good. . . . We will aggressively pursue our search for another and much younger donor."

Since that conversation, I've been in a kind of Limbo, waiting and hoping to hear some positive news from Stanford, and wondering what they might be telling you (hence my sad lack of communication). It was apparent that their MD had serious reservations about my being a donor. I can't say I wasn't relieved by the thought of being spared the procedure but it didn't come without a sinking feeling of letting you down.

Stanford plays their patient confidentiality cards pretty close to their vest, but if my sense of the situation is correct and you're able to pull off another remission, they will have found you a younger donor by then.

Wherever this ultimately ends, there is certainly no lack of love coming from me, and I am looking forward to a future, which holds more hope than fear.

From my heart to you,

Paul

Just like that, I learn it's possible to disagree with someone and still respect them. Life is easier when you can write people off. It's work to have friends with differing opinions—valuable, sure, but also a pain in the ass. People can grow apart, be fundamentally different, and still remain close, like old friends. Like brothers.

I understand now that Paul was in an impossible spot, similar to Dad's. Though he wasn't risking death, the dilemma was the same. He was on a ledge, too. Behind him was the villainous disease threatening to kill his brother. Below him, the uncertainty of a transplant, something he considered voodoo science, a toe in the ritual stew. He stalled on that ledge, waiting, hoping, looking behind him, then down, then back and down again. In the last minute, he was rescued. Dad, on the other hand, will have to jump.

Footnotes

Chipping away the January ice with a garden hoe so the neighborhood kids don't have to summit a graying mountain of winter effluvium on their way to school, I get a text from Dad:

Dad
Just got off the phone with Dr. The news is bad. Call me.

The onslaught of toxins still hadn't killed Dad's cancer—that fucking cockroach, tiptoeing through the postapocalyptic shell of his insides. Now that he has failed intensive chemotherapy, his leukemia is "refractory," a high-risk subtype that is stubborn and unresponsive to treatment.

Dr. Levine says that, while some options remain, all of them are long shots, and the likelihood that Dad will die from an infection outweighs the "single-digit percentage" that any heroic measures will result in a sustainable, transplant-worthy remission. "We're looking at months now," he says. Dr. Levine suggests that the next step should be palliative care: transfusions, and timid, less-risky medications aimed not at a cure, but rather at improving the quality of the time that remains.

Dad is torn between his faith in science and deference for his doctor. This is the first time they haven't been in agreement; Dad wants to keep trying for a cure. I don't want him to give up and do nothing (which is arguably doing something), but I fear bearing any responsibility for a decision that could cause him misery in his final months.

A morbid longing for the worst-case scenario leads me back to the Internet: an "off" switch for hope. I learn that treatment of refractory AML is considered "salvage therapy," a last-ditch effort to scavenge the footnotes of medicine. *Let me see if I have something in the shed out back that can fix you.* For obvious reasons, doctors don't use the word "salvage" with patients. It's something found only in medical journals, and, unfortunately, Google's algorithm does not include a variable called "user_is_better_off_not_knowing."

I text Dad's ex-student Doug the news. He responds quickly.

Doug
OK, so what's the next step?

Jason
I don't think there is one, at least not in my dad's opinion or those of his doctor.

Doug
What about a trial? I thought the doc said something about that before.

Jason
Levine tends to be a downer and my Dad is feeling depressed about all this.

Dad is not stubborn. Not anymore. He listens to me. He shouldn't, but he does. I'm glad Doug's stance on this is strong. His refusal to accept the lack of curative options infuses me with enough confidence to stumble my way through a phone call with Dad.

"Jace, you're the expert here. What should I do?" he asks.

"I'm not an expert."

He doesn't believe I am, but he knows that complimenting me will boost my confidence and make me more forthcoming. We use this trick on each other all the time. We're both cognizant of when the other is employing it, and neither of us cares.

"Well, you know more than I do," he says.

"None of the science matters," I say. "You have to decide what you want."

"I want those boys to have a grandpa," he says.

"Me, too. So there's really only one option."

Dad is fully capable of drawing a straight line between two points. The man knows how to install a toilet flusher. He's read *Das Kapital*—all of it—multiple times. Who the hell does that? Clearly, he knows that to be cured, he will have to take this bet. He doesn't need an expert. He needs someone to tell him it can work, and even if it doesn't, that he's doing the right thing.

An hour later, he texts me:

Dad
You have convinced me. I will not go gentle into that good night.

Jason
Goddamn right.

Dad
Thanks for not letting me give up.

Dad chose long ago to fight this, and though he is losing, there's always a chance, however slight, that one lucky, flailing punch will land squarely on his opponent's chin. I share his doubt, but it's my job to massage his shoulders, offer him sips of water, rub that weird jelly shit on his cheekbones, and spank him on the ass.

But Dad is tired, emotionally drained, and so am I. A heart attack, stroke, parachute failure: something devoid of all these peaks and valleys might have been easier. Had this been an event, Dad would have been dead for over a year by then, and we would have started the process of moving on. Or I would be on lithium. Or I'm naïve and terrible at predicting things. My point is, I would be somewhere. Chipping all this ice and feeling proud that I transformed a mountain into an icy knoll only reminds me of what little progress I've made toward accepting the specter of Dad's mortality. Wouldn't it have been easier for all of us to skip this part and go straight to accepting that he's gone?

———

Clinical trials are more or less experiments, conducted only at teaching hospitals. Stanford is the best in the Bay Area. I have been scanning the government databases, looking for new fancy stuff Dad can try, but find it hard to discern whether some wacky combination of traditional chemo and cholesterol-lowering drugs might work for him, or if he would even be a candidate. Like prep schools, one must apply, interview, and be accepted to a clinical trial. Rather than tests of knowledge and achievement, applicants are selected based on their likelihood to survive.

After Dad makes contact with a researcher at Stanford, Doug flies his airplane to Palo Alto to attend the meeting with him. He records the conversation and emails it to me. The principle investigator of the trial concurs with Dr. Levine: any treatment at this point is a long shot. But he seems eager to include Dad. Maybe a little too eager, like a college booster wooing a high school basketball phenom. Of course, their intentions are pure: they want to help people, and they need patients who are out of options. Still, the phrase "recruiting volunteers" leaves us feeling a bit Tuskegee Airmen about the whole thing. But thinking his only other choice is going gently into that good night, Dad agrees to enter the trial.

For insurance purposes, he has to obtain Dr. Levine's approval. When Dad contacts him, he acts as if we'd called his bluff. He tells Dad *not* to do the trial, that it seems "far-fetched," and says that if Dad insists on further treatment, there's something more established he can try. There is, as it turns out, a protocol for "salvage chemotherapy" located in the main text of medical science, not in the footnotes.

Despite the fact that Dad's first round of intensive chemotherapy was unsuccessful, he still made his way through without so much as running a fever. Why not try again by adding a newer chemotherapy drug and increasing the doses of the others? No matter how stubborn his leukemia, it has to respond to something.

Dr. Levine schedules Dad to go in the next day for a new treatment. I offer to come out, but since he's been through it once before, Dad knows the drill and encourages me to stay home with my family. "We can FaceTime four times a day if we want," he says. "Plus, Mom and Doug will be nearby to come visit."

Lindsay expresses concern about how I might react should something go wrong. She looks at me sternly. "I just want to make sure that if you get a phone call from your mom telling you that your dad is about to die, that you'll be okay with not having been there."

"Hell no, I won't be okay with that. I'm only four hours away. If there's an emergency, I can catch the next flight out."

"Right," she says, unconvinced. "Just don't stay here because of me. I'll be fine here by myself with the kids."

"I know. I'll be fine. He'll be fine. Honestly, I think he doesn't want this whole thing to take over my life anymore."

In fact, I'd been having a difficult time. My mental state had become too dependent on Dad's condition, and distance, as odd as it feels to us, is probably the best thing. And it took some distance, both physical and emotional, for Dad and me realize that our circumstances may have control over what we *do*, but they do not dictate how we feel or what we talk about. Letting go of the idea that somehow we can control the future enables us to appreciate our time in a manner that isn't structured by a morbid fascination with his illness or the jelly-beaned hope that it will disappear.

Jason
You nervous?

Dad
Not so much. It's an either/or situation and I know pretty much what to expect in either case.

Jason
Same here. Oddly calm about it.

Dad
I think we might have both exhausted our anxiety for a time.
How's everyone there in the cold land?

Jason
40 degrees here today! I'm wearing just a fleece.

<u>Dad</u>
Snow all gone?

<u>Jason</u>
Oh God no.

<u>Dad</u>
What are you guys doing today?

<u>Jason</u>
Silas and I are bowling.

<u>Dad</u>
That's adorable.

Dad is ready to start moving on, to stop talking incessantly about his disease and treatment, but I'm not quite there yet. Later that night, while feeling powerless and without anything specific to worry about, I turn to my trusted enabler: the Internet. I discover that the most common source of infection while receiving chemo doesn't come from the outside environment—or even from inside the hospital via an errant hack from a neighboring patient with tuberculosis—it comes from the bacteria and viruses already living inside our bodies. I was unaware that each of us walks around in a constant state of fighting ourselves, that our healthy immune systems are always shooing away the gnats of disease. Finally, an answer as to why I'm so tired all the time.

The next morning at around 8 AM, as I cut the crusts off a peanut-butter-and-honey sandwich for Silas's lunch, and Lindsay explains to Arlo why he can't put paprika on his bowl of Puffins, I get a text from Mom:

Mom
OK, now don't panic.

Luckily, my brain was running dangerously low on panic juice.

Jason
What's going on?

Mom
Dad has what they think is tonsillitis. He's OK, but here's the number of the doctor on staff if you want to talk to her . . .

Jason
I'll call and let you know what I find out.

Mom knows I will want more details than she can provide. Having been at this for over a year, we try not to speculate anymore. The circular Q&As always end with Dad saying, "Well, none of us know what the hell we're talking about here, do we?"

I talk to doctors the same way I talk to the "geniuses" at the Apple store. I want answers, but I also want to show them that I'm smart and fluent in their language. "Well, I updated to the latest firmware, then did a full restore, and I'm still having the problem. I'd say it's a hardware rather than a software issue, right?" With doctors, I like to think that my history as a hypochondriac provides me with at least an honorary medical degree. I also don't like wasting their time. But most of all, when I call the hospital, I don't want to hear the "What cancer is" or "How the immune system works" speeches again.

After spraying my hose of armchair oncology on the doctor—one that probably sounds to her like a person speaking French for the first time after spending a month with Rosetta Stone—she tells me not to worry. "This is common," she says. "Almost everyone going through this kind of treatment gets an infection at some point. Compared to all the other things your father could have contracted, this is tame. And he's already responding to the antibiotics."

I am still breathing heavily in anticipation of some sweet follow-up questions, but can't think of any. She aced her response, and all I can muster is "Thank you very much" and "It was nice of you to take the time to talk to me." I imagine her smirking. No, she isn't thinking about *me* at all.

I call Dad to let him know what I found. It is still heroic to him that I talk to physicians on the telephone, and I need an ego boost.

"Hewwo?" The voice on the other end is husky and muddled like a career smoker with an enlarged tongue.

"Dad?"

"Hey, Dace."

"Jesus, you sound like Mickey Rourke."

I can barely understand him, but am able to gather that his throat was nearly swollen shut and the nurses had given him morphine for the pain. That's two strikes against speaking clearly.

He emails me thirty minutes later, saying he feels better than he sounds and that if the doctors aren't worried, I shouldn't be.

A few minutes later, Doug texts me.

Doug
I texted your dad and he never got back to me. Everything OK?

I tell him about the infection, which he takes in stride. Doug's good at not worrying about things that shouldn't worry him. A hippie turned entrepreneur, he's also adept at ignoring troubling issues, but that's not the case here. We continue texting, and become a bit wistful. We decided that when Dad's time comes, we will pool funds (mostly his) to rename Elliot Hall (the old colonial that's home to the Politics and Government Department at Ohio Wesleyan) after Dad: "Good Hall" or "The Michael Good School of Politics." Neither has a ring to it, but such is the fate of having an adjective for a last name.

I always wanted a big brother, and though Doug never shows up for Christmas, doesn't call regularly, and wasn't present during my childhood, he loves my dad. By extension, I imagine he loves me, too. I tell him that he's "like my big brother now." "Cool," he responds. "I never liked being the youngest anyway." It's the perfect masculine response: a funny but unsweetened confirmation of a shared emotion.

Thinking it might brighten him, I tell Dad of our plans to rename Elliot Hall. I should have known that he would have no interest.

"That's sweet, but also a tremendous waste of money," he says.

"Then we'll do it for us."

"If that's what you want."

It's difficult to accept that the world continues after you die. I'm sure Dad doesn't want to talk about how things might be when he's gone. I thought I was being altruistic and loving, but realized it was nothing more than a projection of my own coping. He'd already made his wishes clear: "I won't want or need anything when I'm dead." No funeral, no sprinkling of his ashes from the Palazzo Vecchio, no token of his legacy at Ohio Wesleyan. He has never wavered in that, but how can he be *so sure*?

The morning after our casino win in Egypt in 1992, we visited the Valley of the Kings. With our little tourist map of the ancient burial grounds in hand, we wandered from tomb to tomb. The pharaohs were unanimous: dead people need shit—some myrrh, maybe a statue missing half its face, perhaps a listless cat. I was twenty (a deceptively impressionable age) and for the subsequent two years I wore an ankh around my neck. Not only did I think it was a hilarious addition to my six-inch-long goatee, it was also a little insurance policy in case the Egyptians were on to something. When it's my time to die, I'll probably request that Silas and Arlo put a boat next to my urn, in case I have a long journey down the River Styx ahead of me. Like Dad says about prayer, it can't hurt.

Humankind has come a long way in five thousand years. Contemporary spirituality suggests that upon death, the energy of the soul transfers to other organisms. In your body right now—yes, right this very moment—are atoms and molecules that were once inside Thomas Jefferson, or a mastodon, perhaps a lonely sycamore tree, or any millions of random organic things, including Genghis Khan. Cool thought, but who cares, really? What does that leave for us survivors? A fern can't make me laugh. Most horses can't tell me I'm full of shit. And no other human being can imitate an old Jewish man saying "celery" quite like Dad.

Hinterland

"Do you have a sword?"

"Huh?" I answer, busy searching for a torch on the other half of the screen.

"Do. You. Have. A. Sword." I think Silas wants a sword. He's become far better at this video game than I.

"Oh yeah, I have one. Sorry, I was over in that cage trying to find a torch."

"We don't need a torch," he says, incredulous. What kind of rube would look for a torch in this situation? I like it when my six-year-old son treats me like an idiot.

"Come over here so we can use the cannon," he says.

"Okay, boss. I'm coming. Wait, where are you?"

"Over here."

"Where?"

"Whatever. Can I just be you?"

"Sure." I switch controllers with him.

He inserts the sword into a slot to activate the cannon. His half of the screen zooms in to show the target. He aims at the opposing ship. We have to hit it three times, I think.

"There. Right there!" I shout.

He fires. "Yes!"

"Nice shot, bud! Hey, do you remember what I told you about Boo-Boo getting new blood?" I ask. I mean stem cells, but I never explained the details of Dad's transplant to him. Mostly because I'm incapable.

"Yes. Is he getting it?" Silas aims the cannon again.

"He is."

"Darn!" He misses. "So, his brother's blood will make him not sick anymore?"

"He's not getting it from his brother."

"Why not?"

"They decided he's too old."

"Ugh!" He misses again. "Daddy, can you do it?" We switch controllers, and I aim up.

"You hit it!" he shouts. "Who's he getting it from, then?

"The blood? From someone he doesn't know."

"And he's getting it right now?" Silas asks.

"No, not for a few weeks."

"So he'll get it while we're there?"

"No. We're going there tomorrow, you doofus. You know that. Here, do you want to do the last one?" We switch controllers again.

He hits the ship, and it starts to sink. We jump in the rowboat and start making our way over. I'm nervous. We have to get there before it becomes submerged or . . .

Lindsay walks in. "Hey, guys."

"Hi," we respond, still cyber-rowing.

"Remember, Silas," she says, "you're only allowed to play Wii for thirty minutes on weekdays."

"Oh, he knows," I say, staring at the screen. "I have the timer going. There's still ten more minutes."

"Great." She tries to make eye contact with Silas. "You have homework to do after this."

"Yeah, yeah," he mumbles. I kick his foot. He sits up straight and looks his mother in the eye. "Okay, Mommy."

When she walks out, Silas glances over at me.

I wink at him. "Let's just keep going until we finish the level."

"But what about the timer?"

"It's close enough."

He smiles and turns his attention back to the game. "So when is BooBoo going to get better?"

"If it works, six months."

"But he's not going to die?"

"We still don't know."

"Daddy! We can use the girl to jump on top of that thing."

"The sea monster?"

"Yeah!"

After the boys fall asleep, Lindsay and I do our postmortem for the day.

"I really want to stick by this half an hour of Wii on weekdays thing," she says. "I just read an article saying that kids should only look at screens for a maximum of one hour a day."

"And he's allowed to watch one half-hour TV show after school, right?" I ask.

"Yes. Wait, how do you not know that?"

"I do. I'm encouraging you to do the math."

"Right. Just don't let it be more than thirty minutes of Wii. I hate screens. Kids should be outside all the time like I was at his age."

"I stare at screens for probably 90 percent of the time I'm awake, and there's another 5 percent of the day that I spend searching for my phone. And look how I'm turning out."

She laughs. "Are you packed yet?"

"No. All our devices are charged, though."

"Both iPads?"

"Yup."

"Okay, good."

On March 31, we flew from Minneapolis to San Francisco. On the plane ride, Silas and I split the cracked pepper turkey sandwich. Across the aisle, Lindsay and Arlo share a fruit and cheese plate. The kids are calm. Silas watches *The Incredibles* on one iPad; Arlo, *Peter Rabbit* on the other. I play Guitar Hero on my phone, and Lindsay is deep into Temple Run on hers.

We don't know if this trip is going to be a good-bye for Dad and his grandsons, Lindsay, and me. His chances are only 50/50 that the transplant will cure him, but I feel differently than I did last November. And so does he. We all do. After Dad's first remission, I believed that as long as he made it to the transplant, he would go all the way. Perhaps I'm merely breaking our journey into manageable chunks, and this is nothing more than the sensation one has after taking a beautiful piss during a road-trip pit stop. We are at a juncture—somewhere above Barstow, on the edge of the desert, but at least we're pointed in the direction of Las Vegas.

The salvage chemotherapy that was unlikely to work, worked. The roulette wheel spun until we bit our fingers raw, but when it stopped, the croupier shoved a big stack of chips in front of Dad and said, "Congratulations, sir. If you wish to continue playing, please take these over to the high-stakes tables."

He got lucky. But over the past couple of months, I have stopped hoping. I wouldn't say I lost it, though. My hope merely rolled under the bed, fell between the sofa cushions, or lodged itself in the junk drawer. It's somewhere, but I'm no longer looking, because when it left, fear went with it.

Now, when I imagine Dad dying, I see very specific images, and I can almost feel what it would be like to see those images with my eyes and not just my mind. I prepare for a jolt of panic, but it doesn't come anymore. My brain has been practicing. Sure, there's sadness, and something I can only describe as "weirdness," but unless those emotions are accompanied by "Cat's in the Cradle" by Harry Chapin or "Skating Away" by Jethro Tull (which, admittedly, I listen to in excess), they're not overwhelming, and even then, they evaporate quickly under the hot sun of my life with Lindsay and the boys.

I'm here for them again. Not because I finished something, but rather because that something finished with me. Seeking hope and enduring fear is hard, even brave, but maybe what has gotten me through in the end is finally facing this situation with neither. I'm not sure how one does that, because, for me, it was unwitting. But I do know that you can't thread a piece of spaghetti through a crazy straw without cooking it first. And then, I imagine it's not easy.

The idea that I could control what was happening to Dad, or control how I deal with what is happening to him, to us, seems to have vanished. I thought I was holding on in error, but maybe I was keeping it all close, nurturing it, feeding the parasite of pregrief until it pushed away from the dinner table, wiped its mouth, and asked to borrow sweatpants. I never thought I was *feeling* appropriately. I was either too sad or not sad enough, too involved or too distant. Everyone works through something like this differently. The problem is, we don't know in advance exactly what our way might be. Without accurate expectations, experiences will always feel a bit foreign. Perhaps life would be boring if everything went as planned. How California of me.

After landing in Oakland, the four of us make the same walk we did a year and a half ago. We bought Arlo his own suitcase, to put him on equal luggage footing with his older brother.

In the BART station, on the same platform where I threw a tantrum over a year ago, Lindsay is the tense parent this time. "Arlo, stop running! The train is coming soon," she says.

"Arlo, come over here," Silas adds, trying to help.

"That's the same voice you use when you're talking to one of our cats," I tell him.

I make a kissing sound. "Arlo, do you want a treat?" Silas thinks it's hilarious.

When Arlo sees the train approaching, he runs over to us and grabs the handle of his miniature suitcase. Good kitty.

Mom and Dad don't meet us at the station this time. The boys complain that their bags are too heavy, so Lindsay carries Arlo's and I carry Silas's.

Mom and Dad answer the door. They couldn't be happier that we're all here. In the kitchen, I notice that half of the wine refrigerator has been delegated to various flavors of Ensure.

While Mom shows Arlo the new box of Play-Doh she bought him, and Lindsay unpacks with Silas, Dad and I sit in the living room.

On the coffee table, there's a thick folder with a photograph on the cover displaying people of various ages and ethnicities—all of them smiling. "What to Expect from Your Transplant" it's titled, in a cheerful font.

I pick it up and glance at Dad. "Did you read this?"

"Some of it," he says.

"Should I read it?"

"Nah."

I toss it back on the table as if folding a hand of poker. It stays there, unopened, for five days. In the mornings, Lindsay, Mom, Dad, and I use it as a coaster for our coffee. In the afternoons, Mom and Silas play cards on it.

The boys tromp back into the living room and plop down on the sofa next to BooBoo. Dad puts his arms around them, and squeezes. "Ah, my number one and number two boys." They smile, and Dad yells, "Hello??? Can I get a picture here?" Lindsay, Mom, and I get in line, and the boys both smile. Dad's hair has grown back into an adorable little faux-hawk, and he looks like one of those old guys in New York who was never able to give up the punk movement.

Later, Dad and I take the boys to Marina Park. It is a bit cold, but we all get Popsicles anyway. Silas completes the monkey bars without assistance for the first time, and then he and Arlo climb on the rocky beach as we watch. After a few minutes, our gazes turn to a nice boat tied up to the dock.

"Someday," he says.

"Someday soon," I respond. We aren't even boat people, but if there is a future, it's wide open. Maybe we'll have a scotch together, my first in eight years. I imagine we might crank some Vivaldi, slump down in matching white leather chairs, and sip slowly from highball glasses, like a couple of Hollywood antiheroes after spoiling an evil plot.

When we arrive back in the apartment, Silas parks himself in front of the television in Dad's den. He knows how to work all the remotes. Arlo wanders off, but soon comes running back to the living room, where the rest of us sit. "Bozo won't stand up," he says. I get up to investigate and find that Arlo has put our punching bag out of its misery with a pencil to the groin. Mom tries to fix the hole with duct tape, but Bozo will never fully recover.

Arlo joins Silas in the den. The boys are tired, and so is Dad. So am I. I feel five years older than I did a year and a half ago. I now use ointments and creams daily. I feel the need to compensate, but since I can't afford a 1957 Camaro SS, I bought an electronic drum set instead. I put on headphones and play along to Rush, like the character Nick on *Freaks and Geeks*, except Nick was in high school. Sometimes I smoke my e-cig while playing my e-drums. I'm an e-person now: a cyborg of science fiction's boring daydreams. I'm settled with who I am, I guess. I've demolished and rebuilt temporary housing. I tossed the peach-flavored e-cigs and replaced them with a new brand, with new flavor options. I chose Absolute Tobacco because it's manly, confident, and unafraid.

Maybe that mortar I once felt in my brain, and the brick wall it held together, wasn't there to block anything or to help me cope. Nor was it indicative of avoidance or turning off. Maybe it was a symbol of completion. Or maybe it was never there at all. That therapist was right to encourage me to trust my process. I still believe that not trusting my process is an integral part of my process, but if I can feel assured that self-doubt serves me, maybe I'll stop questioning it so much.

I still don't know how I will react if the transplant doesn't work and Dad dies. This pregrief stuff doesn't come with a guarantee, just as pregame tailgating doesn't guarantee that your favorite team will win or that you won't spend the first quarter in the bathroom, sick from the three bratwursts you consumed at 9 AM in the parking lot.

My sons are getting older. Silas is asserting his independence, and Arlo is in an astonishingly cute phase, but I know we can't keep him there for long. I was fifteen when Dad was my age. I couldn't understand him then, mostly because I was still a mystery to myself. But I remember what he wore, how he smelled, the rhythm of his snore, how he put his socks on before his pants. When Silas is fifteen, I'll be fifty-one: an age that can go either way. I've seen fit, spritely fifty-somethings, with young men's eyes, and I've seen others with nothing left, who spend all their days searching the hardware store, grimacing, not quite knowing what they're looking for. Maybe spot cleaner for the fake grass on their back porch? Bungee cords? A chainsaw? Anything to make themselves feel useful.

The duration of our confluence has lasted longer than Dad and I expected. It might, in fact, have run its natural course (whatever that means). I would undo the circumstances of the last eighteen months if I could, but had Dad not gotten sick—if he had instead dropped suddenly from a rage-induced heart attack at Radio Shack—we might not have been alerted that it was happening. We could have missed the eclipse entirely or found out too late and not had enough time to make our cardboard viewing box.

On April 20, Dad checked into the Stanford Medical Center for prepara-
tory chemotherapy to kill his white blood cells again. His marrow has
had only a month to actualize any nefarious plans, and I almost feel sorry
for it. It's like that moment toward the end of every Disney movie when
you sympathize with the villain only to shake it off when you remember
all of the terrible things he has done.

Dad is hooked up to the poison, and his new stem cells are on the
way: the seeds of a new beginning. A frozen bag of beige stuff floating
thirty thousand feet above the Great Lakes, or over the ocean, or a corn-
field. We don't know where it's coming from. We only know the donor
is a fifty-seven-year-old male. We aren't permitted to know any other
information about him for three years.

I'll be visiting Dad when he gets out of the hospital. We decided
I don't need to come for the transplant. He emails me a cute little calen-
dar the nurses made for him. Written in the April 20 box is "Transplant"
and "Happy Birthday!!!"

I email him back. "Wow, and it's on your birthday! How amazing
is that?"

"No, my birthday is on the twenty-fourth," he writes.

I didn't know that transplant day is referred to as the patient's
birthday. Apparently, I also don't know the date of my father's actual
birthday. I know it's somewhere in the 20-somethings of April. I'm a good
son. I'm just not good with dates. I know Mom's birthday is somewhere
between May 12 and May 16. They never made me feel guilty for not
knowing and I don't do anything unless badgered. Lindsay's birthday is
March 22.

Dad

They just told me my blood type will change after the transplant.

Jason

That's weird. Makes sense though now that I think about it. Does that technically change your ethnicity to that of the donor?

Dad

Hadn't thought of that.

Jason

If the guy is Native American, maybe you can start raking in some sweet casino money.

Dad

Depends on which tribe he's in.

Jason

Ha.

Dad

I won't have any immunities either and will have to be revaccinated for everything. MMR, Polio, etc.

Jason

Also weird. Do you go to a pediatrician for those?

Dad

No, they do them here.

I was kidding.

Dad
I know.

Jason
What if they make you autistic?

Dad
I'll take it.

Jason
Holy shit. Read this thing I just found on the web: "The preserving agent used when freezing the donor's stem cells causes many of these side effects. You might have a strong taste of garlic or creamed corn in your mouth."

Dad
Now I'm hungry.

Jason
Haha. That's a liberal definition of side effect. Whoa, ever more bizarre. From the same site: "Your body will also smell like this. The smell may bother those around you, but you might not even notice it. The smell, along with the taste, may last for a few days, but slowly fades away. Often having cut up oranges in the room will offset the odor."

After 25 minutes, Dad responded:

<u>Dad</u>
I feel like this is going to work.

<u>Jason</u>
Me too.

———

One summer day when I was eleven, Mom, Dad, and I had plans to go to the zoo. For the previous three weeks, however, I had been pilfering quarters from Dad's change bowl and burying them in Mom's flower bed next to the front porch (perhaps this was overly cautious). That morning, I'd decided to dig up my treasure and head to the Electric Animal and Screen Door—a video arcade located on the meager downtown strip in Delaware. It was filled with twenty-somethings gambling on games of Joust, Q*bert, and Frogger, their lighted cigarettes balancing on the edge, burning brown lines into the plastic casings. Dad had forbidden me from going there, but it was seedy, and that made me want to go all the more. So I did, every weekend, and always under the ruse of going for a bike ride. Mom and Dad must have thought I was becoming such a wholesome boy, tootling around for hours on my turd-colored Schwinn. With little money of my own, I normally watched the older guys play, but on this morning, I had a couple pounds of dirty quarters stuffed in the pockets of my corduroy shorts.

When I arrived at 10 AM, there was a tear in space-time. Instead of watching others, I played the games now. At around 1 PM, while abusing the joystick of Dig Dug, I was startled by an aggressive tap on my shoulder. I whipped around to find Dad standing behind me. His face was red, hair slick from anger sweat. I immediately started crying—not out of fear (though there was some of that)—but more out of guilt. I wanted a do-over, to stay home and watch TV in the morning and enjoy the zoo as a family later.

Dad pulled me out by my elbow, picked up my bike, threw it in the back of our Plymouth Volaré, and drove us home in silence. On the front porch, I wiped the tear residue from my cheeks as Mom and Dad leered at me. "So all these *bike rides*—every single goddamn one of them—you were really going to that arcade?" Dad asked. Mom frowned at me.

"No!" I lied. "Only some of them. And I only ever watched. I mean, until today."

"I don't care what you *did* there. I didn't say you weren't allowed to play video games. I said you weren't allowed to go to that rancid place."

"I didn't know that!" I said, sensing an easy way out.

"Oh bullshit. You knew that. I don't care about you playing video games. I don't want you hanging around people with dirty T-shirts and hockey hair." Dad paused for a moment, then continued, "Jesus Christ, it's almost worse that you watched. Who watches someone play a video game? How bored do you have to be to watch someone do something that's already boring?"

His anger turned to disbelief, which triggered his comedic imagination. "What is it that you *do*, exactly, while watching these guys? Do you talk to them? Tell them, 'Nice move, buddy'? Get them sodas? Are you some kind of corner man for them? Jesus Christ, Jason."

We sat in silence, each of us staring off into a separate distance. I think Dad felt adequately vented, and since it appeared to have been a hot, short fire, I didn't want to reignite it by saying something stupid.

But after a few minutes, I summoned a measure of bravery and asked, "Can we still go to the zoo?" My voice cracked a bit. I wanted nothing more than for things to go back to normal. I suddenly hated that arcade, hated myself for going, and hated my bike and the flower beds for facilitating it all. I wanted to take a sledgehammer to a Dig Dug machine. I think Dad saw this, and after taking a moment, he broke into a smile. "Hell, yes. Let's go to the zoo."

Acknowledgments

To all the people who never lost patience with me:

My mother, Jody Good, who read every word of this book—sometimes sentence by sentence as I emailed them to her, asking, "Is this any good?" She never gave me enough praise so that I'd settle, and never so much criticism that I'd give up.

My father, Michael Good, who is my biggest fan. And I am his. Most sons can't say that about their dads, and I consider myself beyond fortunate.

My wife, Lindsay Forsythe, who orchestrated her own life so that I could write this book. It's what loving spouses do for each other, and I will return the favor whenever she sees fit.

Daniel Smith, Henry Cherry, and Todd Pruzan, who provided the kind of guidance one expects of true friends.

My sons, Silas and Arlo, who know how to live in the moment. To them, there is nothing else. Thank you for always being you, guys.

My writer's group—Stephanie Ash, Geoff Herbach, Mary Mack, and Dennis Cass—somehow made this process more fun than I'd anticipated.

My editor, Lorena Jones, and agent, Courtney Miller-Callihan, who always made time for me and always knew what to say. And to designer Jennifer Tolo Pierce and managing editor Sara Golski for adding polish.

All my other full and partial readers—Amy Bass, Kate Bolick, Emily Chenoweth, Robert Dowling, Carly Kimmel, David Maclean, Virginia Snyder, Dave Toht, Betony Toht, and Amy Williams—whose help I needed. I promise never to be quite so needy again. Unless, of course, I write another book.

Remember when you were young and you thought your dad was Superman, and then you grew up and realized he's just a drunk who wears a cape?

—DAVE ATTELL